Choose this not that

for

Ulcers

by

Personal Remedies

Published by Simple Software Publishing.

Copyright © 2014 by Personal Remedies, LLC
5 Oregon Street
Georgetown, MA 01833 USA

ISBN-13: 978-1494962371   ISBN-10: 1494962373

Printed by CreateSpace.

Choose this not that

for

Ulcers

Inside this book, you will find a list of food items and easy to follow suggestions on how to improve your health through nutrition and the food choices you make every day.

Suggestions are provided for those with Ulcers (Peptic Ulcer) or those who are prone to develop this condition. The term Ulcers is commonly used to describe Peptic Ulcer, while the term ulcer can refer to any form of internal or external wound.

In addition, the book contains similar information for those who have one of the following common health conditions, risks or a diet preference along with Peptic Ulcer:

- Anemia
- Cancer risk
- Depression
- Diabetes (Type 2)
- Excess body weight or obesity
- High Blood Pressure
- High cholesterol
- Menopause
- Stress
- Vitamin D deficiency

Table of Contents

Important Notes

The purpose of this book is to provide helpful and informative material and to educate. It is in no way intended as substitute for medical advice. We recommend in all cases that you contact your personal doctor or health care provider before you embark upon any new diet or treatment of yourself.

This book is sold with the understanding that the publisher, the author and the distributor of this book are neither liable, nor have responsibility to any person or entity with respect to any loss, damage or injury which is incurred as a consequence, directly or indirectly, of the use or application of any of the contents of this book.

How to use this book

The guidelines presented on the following pages are for an adult male or female. They do not apply to children, pregnant women or breast feeding mothers.

Our suggestions are organized by food groups. Within each food group, **items are presented in a specific and deliberate order**. In the case of recommended items (those that could <u>improve</u> your health), the most helpful remedies or suggestions are presented first. In the case of items to avoid (those that could <u>worsen</u> your conditions), the most critical ones to avoid are listed first. The items that are suggested under <u>Instead Choose</u>, or items that are not included in the previous two lists, are likely to be neutral for your health (i.e., neither improve nor worsen your conditions) based on the information available to us at the time.

Unfortunately, health issues often come our way in groups of two or more. If we are obese or under stress, then chances are we are also at risk with a number of other health issues such as cancer, high blood pressure, or Vitamin D deficiency. If we have Vitamin D deficiency then chances are we either suffer from or have higher risk of getting Osteoporosis, Crohn's disease or kidney problems. Each health issue often results in other health complications, thus the need for looking at a combination of health concerns and risks when formulating our nutrition plans and lifestyle changes. It is for that reason, that we have included separate guidelines for those who might suffer from the most likely and common combinations of health issues related to the main health concern addressed by this book.

One of the factors that make *Choose this not that* series of publications different from all others available to you in the market is that we offer nutrition guidelines for likely COMBINATIONS of illnesses and risks that may be relevant to your situation. We also give you specific guidance by telling you exactly which fish, fruit, vegetable, nut … is the best for you as well as listing the worst items. We give you an ordered list of food items within each food group, not just a food group.

We have listed alternative therapies and herbal medicines relevant (either helpful or harmful) to your condition. But it is beyond the scope of this book to provide specific guidelines on dosage or how to best benefit from these options. We encourage you to explore these alternatives with your natural health care provider.

Our approach in the *Choose this not that* series is to help people improve or combat their health issues through nutrition (i.e., consumption of food items that they can easily find in their local grocery store), exercise and lifestyle changes. We accomplish that through identification of those items that can improve your health, those that can worsen it, and those that play a neutral role. We trust that you can use this information to alter your diet and lifestyle choices to improve your health and wellbeing.

How we developed the content of this book

To provide specific and actionable information and guidance on food choices that you make every day and how they might impact your health, we had to quantify a relative level of goodness (or badness) for every individual food item in our database as they relate to each specific illness or health concern tracked in our system.

Most food and nutrition related research and publications in the U.S. are focused on vitamins, minerals, micro-nutrients, and substances such as cholesterol, fat and fiber. And to a lesser extent there are studies and data on herbal remedies, alternative and complementary medicine, and non-western treatments.

There is very little data or widely accepted studies that focus on individual foods (e.g., watermelon, white fish and walnuts) and how they relate to specific illnesses or health risks. Our goal has been to help address that void.

Here is a very brief description of our approach:

a) We maintain detailed nutrition information on every individual food item in our system. Most of such data is available from the U.S. Department of Agriculture. And for some data (e.g., Mercury, Gluten) we have found other reliable sources.

b) When there is data available on health benefits (or adverse impact) of a specific food item, or nutrient (e.g., vitamins, minerals) we capture and make use of such data.

c) If a given nutrient is good for a health condition (e.g., Vitamin A is good for night blindness), then all food items that are rich in that nutrient (Vitamin A) are given a positive/higher rating as they relate to that condition (night blindness). Similarly if a given nutrient has adverse impact on a health condition then all food items that contain that nutrient are given a negative/lower rating.

d) Some food items contain much more of a nutrient than others. Our technology takes that into account.

e) Some nutrients are found to be much more effective (e.g., Vitamin A) than some other nutrient (e.g., Zinc) as they relate to a given health condition (e.g., night blindness). Our technology distinguishes between the two.

f) Sometimes a study or a source behind the relationship between a nutrient and a health condition is much more reliable than another. Our approach is sensitive to that.

g) Certain nutrients facilitate absorption of another nutrient (e.g., Vitamin D facilitates absorption of Calcium). We make use of such information. For example, let's say Calcium is good for Tooth Development. Then all food items that are rich in Vitamin D are given a more positive consideration as they relate to Tooth Development.

h) Similarly some substances may reduce absorption of or increase the need for another (e.g., Caffeine may increase the need for Calcium). In the above example, all food items that contain Caffeine will receive a negative/lower rating as they relate to Tooth Development.

i) Our process and the steps mentioned above are automated by our unique (proprietary) and patented technology. At the conclusion of our process, there is a single score that represents the level of goodness or badness for every food item as it relates to each health condition maintained in our system. These scores are the basis for all the sorted lists of food items that you find in the Choose This Not That series of publications.

j) For multiple conditions, the sum of these scores is what drives the ranking of the food items and our guidelines.

In closing, it is important to note that in these publications we are not making scientific claims, nor do we suggest perfection of our approach. Our goal is to simply provide a significant improvement over status-quo. No human being or health care specialist can properly and fully take into account the enormity, complexity and contradictions inherent in the interrelationships of food, health, genetics, environment, exercise, lifestyle, etc. that affect our wellbeing. We have merely attempted to use the power of technology to provide you much better and more relevant information to maintain healthier living.

Ulcers (Peptic Ulcer)

Peptic ulcer is an open sore typically in the lining of your stomach but sometimes in esophagus and small intestine. Abdominal pain or a burning stomach pain is the most common symptom.

The sore and the pain that accompanies it are due to the damage from the stomach acid that helps with food digestion. The damage occurs when the mucous layer that protects the lining of our stomach is weakened, or when there is an over-production of stomach acid.

The most likely cause for peptic ulcers is an infection from H. Pylori bacterium. H. Pylori lives in the mucous layer that coats our digestive tract and can cause its inflammation. There are antibiotics that are effective in killing this bacterium.

The second most likely cause for peptic ulcers is on-going use of pain killers known as NSAIDs (Non-Steroidal Anti-Inflammatory Drugs) such as aspirin, ibuprofen drugs such as Advil, and others. These drugs (among others) can irritate, inflame or damage the lining of our digestive tract.

While stress, spicy foods, alcohol and smoking can worsen your condition or pain, none of them are the cause for developing a peptic ulcer. Antacids and eating food may offer temporary relief from pain, but the real cure is in healing of the sores.

You are at most risk to develop peptic ulcer if:
- You are infected by H. Pylori (which can spread through unclean food and water, or kissing someone who is infected);
- You are a 60+ years who regularly takes NSAIDs or pain medications for osteoarthritis or other health issues;
- You smoke;
- You drink alcohol (which can worsen your sores, prevent healing, and increase stomach acid production);

Choose these for Ulcers (Peptic Ulcer)

Top 5 items to choose:

Check for H. Pylori infection; Green leafy vegetables; Cabbage juice; Manuka honey; Slippery Elm (herbal med);

Food items and actions that could improve your health (within a food group, most helpful items are listed first):

Meat, Fish & Poultry

Alaskan king crab; Spiny lobster; Oysters; Pork/Lamb/Veal liver; Chicken heart; Veal shank; Dungeness crab; Abalone;

Eggs, Beans, Nuts and Seeds

Pine nuts; Soy milk; Split peas; Chia seeds; Soybean seeds; Flaxseed; Almonds; Fava beans; Sunflower seeds; Soybeans (green); Safflower seeds; Hazelnuts or Filberts; Green peas; Alfalfa sprouts; Breadnut tree seeds; Peanuts; Cashew nuts; Watermelon seeds; Black walnuts; Beans: black, navy, yellow & white; Chickpeas; Lentils; Pistachio nuts; Hyacinth beans; Sesame seeds;

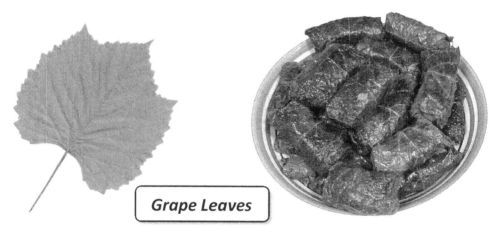

Grape Leaves

Fruits & Juices

Prunes (dried); Kiwi fruit; Dried pears; Blackberries; Dried figs; Passion fruit; Dried peaches; Plantains; Avocado; Dried fruits: Apples, Banana, Apricots; Abiyuch; Boysenberries; Currants (dried); Dates; Elderberries; Guava; Kumquats; various berries; Pomegranate; Raisins; Rhubarb; Rowal; Tamarind; Dried fruits; Olives; Blueberries and Bilberries; Breadfruit; Cranberries; Currants (raw); Durian; Figs; Grapes; Pears; Pomegranate juice; Banana; Acerola; Apple juice; Apples; Apricots; Cantaloupe; Cherries; Cranberry juice; Grape juice; Honeydew melon; Jujube (fruit); Litchi; Longans; Mango; Natal Plum (Carissa); Nectarine; Papaya; Peaches; Persimmons; Pineapple; Pineapple juice; Pitanga; Plum; Prune juice; Quince; Strawberries; Watermelon;

Vegetables

Grape leaves; Shitake mushrooms; Sun-dried tomatoes; Pigeon peas; Sweet potatoes leaves; Dandelion Greens; Green & red cabbages (especially in juice forms); Beet greens; Chicory greens; Collards; Mustard greens; Taro leaves; Turnip greens; Chinese broccoli; Savoy cabbage; Chrysanthemum (Garland); Endive; Fungi cloud ears; Green onions (scallions); Kelp; Ancho & Pasilla peppers; Spinach; Swiss chard; Amaranth leaves; Arugula; Balsam pear leafy tips; Garden cress; Kale; Romaine & loose leaf lettuce; Pokeberry shoots; Watercress; Asparagus; Artichoke; Bok choy; Leeks; Okra; Wasabi root; Parsnips; Jalapeno peppers; Carrots; Celery; Epazote; Green beans; Head lettuce; Taro; Balsam pear; Cauliflower; Chrysanthemum Leaves; Cucumbers with peel; Eggplant; Fennel; Hearts of palm; Kohlrabi; Lotus root; Mustard spinach; Banana pepper; Quinoa seed; Shallots; Sweet potatoes; Winged beans leaves; Yam; Red bell peppers; Broccoli (sprouts in particular); Brussels sprouts; Garlic; Arrowhead; Arrowroot; Jerusalem artichoke; Beets; Green bell peppers; other vegetables;

Breads, Grains, Cereals, Pasta

Rye; Corn bran; Durum wheat; Buckwheat; Whole-wheat; Amaranth; Wheat bran; Whole-wheat cereal; Wheat germ cereal; Whole-wheat bread; Whole-wheat English muffins; Triticale; Whole-wheat spaghetti; Wheat germ; Sorghum; Spelt (cooked); Wheat bran muffins; Barley; Bulgur; Rice bran; Wild rice; Whole-wheat crackers; Oatmeal (cereal); Corn; Millet; Brown rice; Wheat germ bread; Bran flakes cereal; Whole-wheat dinner rolls; Oat bran; Oats;

Dairy Products, Fats & Oils

Yogurt; Wheat germ oil; Canola oil;

Desserts, Snacks, Beverages

Air popped popcorn; Honey (Manuka honey for stomach ulcer in particular); Oil popped popcorn; Sesame crunch candies;

Herbs & Spices, Fast Foods, Prepared Foods

Whole-grain cornmeal; Tofu; Coriander/Cilantro; Parsley; Basil (fresh); Cayenne (red) pepper; Cinnamon (stomach ulcer in particular); Cole slaw; Cottonseed meal; Natto; Thyme (fresh); Tempeh; Maple sugar; Teriyaki sauce; Miso; Rosemary (fresh); Peppermint; Sweet pickle;

Alternative Therapies & Miscellaneous

Consult your doctor (check for H. Pylori infection & if so ask for antibiotics to eliminate); Antacids (to neutralize stomach acid and reduce pain); Elimination diet (need to determine which foods cause problems for you); Biofeedback; Detoxification (3-day juice fast to alkalinize digestive tract); Eat smaller, more frequent meals; Alkaline diet;

Key Nutrients & Herbal Medicines

Slippery Elm (for stomach ulcer in particular); Licorice (use in paste form); Fiber; German chamomile; Irish Moss (taken in a specially prepared commercial form); Vitamin K; Zinc;

Do not choose these for   Ulcers (Peptic Ulcer)

Top 5 items to avoid:

Aspirin & Prescription drugs; Chocolate; Alcoholic beverages; Caffeine; Citrus fruits;

Avoid or consume much less of the following (within a food group, most harmful items are listed first):

Meat, Fish & Poultry

Blood sausage; Pepperoni; Beef & pork frankfurters; Beef & pork luncheon meats; Chorizo; various sausage; Turkey pastrami; Various salami; Pork skins; Chicken skin; Turkey skins; Pork liver cheese; Bacon; Pork breakfast strips;

Instead choose: Blue crab; Cuttlefish; Lobster; Octopus; Beef liver; Beef filet mignon; Beef round steak; Turkey liver; Veal shoulder/leg/sirloin; Ground beef; Anchovy; Snail; Clams; Mussels; Whelk; Chicken & Turkey giblets; Chicken liver; Corned beef; Beef rib eye; Beef top sirloin; Fish roe; Lamb leg; Crayfish; Sardines; Shrimp; Calamari; Carp; Perch; Pout; Pumpkinseed sunfish; Scallops; Smelt; White fish; Boar meat; Quail breast; Rabbit meat; Turkey dark meat; Venison; Chicken breast (no skin); Duck (no skin); Pork cured/ham; Quail; Veal loin; Pork loin/sirloin; Beef; Bison/Buffalo meat; Marlin; Orange roughy; Swordfish; various fish;

Eggs, Beans, Nuts and Seeds

Coconut Milk;

Instead choose: Pecans; Pumpkin & squash seeds; various beans; Black-eyed peas; Sugar or snap peas; Cottonseed; Cornnuts; Lupin; Butternuts; Breadfruit seeds; Chestnuts; Hickory nuts; Ginkgo nuts; Brazil nuts; Walnuts; Coconut meat; Acorns; Beechnuts; Egg white; Egg; Egg substitute;

Fruits & Juices

Grapefruit; Grapefruit juice; Orange juice; Oranges; Pumelo (Shaddock); Tangerines; Lemon; Lime;

Breads, Grains, Cereals, Pasta

Croissant; Danish pastry;

Instead choose: Shredded wheat; Granola cereal; Pumpernickel bread; Oat bran muffins; Rice cakes (Brown rice based); Tortillas (corn); Chinese chow Mein noodles; Toasted bread; Bread sticks; Italian bread; Oat bran bread; English muffins; Corn muffins; Semolina; Wheat; Wheat crackers; Cornbread; Melba toasts crackers; Bagels; Blueberry muffins; Couscous; various noodles; Pasta; White rice; Spaghetti; Banana bread;

Dairy Products, Fats & Oils

Chocolate milk; Milk; Cream cheese; Goat cheese; Cream; Whipped cream; Cheese: Gjetost, limburger, Roquefort; Butter; Cheese spread; various cheese; Sour cream; Lard; Animal fat; Sesame oil; Poultry fat; Whey (dried); Oils: coconut, Cupu Assu, Shea nut, tea seed, Ucuhuba Butter; Oils: cocoa butter, tomato seeds, avocado, mustard; Hydrogenated vegetable oil;

Instead **choose: Margarine; Olive oil; Soybean oil; Margarine-like spreads; Hazelnut oil; Safflower oil; Vegetable shortening; Almonds oil; Grape seeds oil; Apricot kernel oils;**

Desserts, Snacks, Beverages

Sweet chocolate candies; Dark chocolate; Coffee liqueur; Chocolate ice cream; Hot chocolate; 80+ proof distilled alcoholic beverages; Whiskey; Coffee; Chocolate mousse; Crème de menthe; Chocolate chip cookies; Piña colada; Red wine; White wine; Pound cake; Butter cookies; Vanilla ice cream; Dessert toppings; Shortbread cookies; Chocolate (avoid if it bothers you); Plain tea (avoid if it bothers you); various cakes; various cookies; Beer; Frozen yogurt; Milk shakes; After-dinner mints; Cheesecake; Puff pastry; Pudding; Éclairs;

Instead **choose: Tortilla chips; Peanut bar candies; Water; Halvah; Potato chips/fried snacks; Peanut butter; Granola bars; Frostings; Applesauce; Fruit punch; Ginger ale; Lemonade; Sports drinks; Herbal tea; Tonic water; Peanut brittle candies; Hard candies; Marshmallows; Pumpkin pie; Pecan pie;**

Herbs & Spices, Fast Foods, Prepared Foods

Cocoa; Chocolate syrup; Cheese sauce; Horseradish; Mustard seed (avoid if it bothers you); Nutmeg (avoid if it bothers you); Pepper (black or white; avoid if it bothers you); Table sugar (white or powder); Nachos; Foie gras or liver pate; Hot dog; Pizza;

Instead **choose: Fried tofu; Pickle (cucumber); Spearmint (fresh); Tomato paste; Cloves; Oregano; Soy sauce; Cardamom; Croutons; Mayonnaise; Poppy seed; Sage; Sauerkraut; French & Italian salad dressings; French fries; Chervil; Chives; Corn cakes; Egg rolls (veg); Fennel seeds; Hummus; Mace; Mints; Mustard; Pickle relish; Succotash; Maple syrup; Turmeric; Hamburger; Capers; Dill weed; Ginger; Gravies; Marjoram; Saffron; Table salt; Brown sugar; various syrups; Tarragon; Vinegar; various soups & broths; Falafel; Potato pancakes; Cheeseburger; Onion rings; Blue/Roquefort salad dressing;**

Alternative Therapies & Miscellaneous

Aspirin (& other NSAID drugs); Fasting (for a specific period); Prescription drugs (NSAID drugs); Alcoholic beverages; Food allergens (determine if a food allergy triggers your ulcer); Smoking, tobacco; Stress (can worsen your symptoms); Fried or battered foods; Spicy foods;

Key Nutrients & Herbal Medicines

Alcohol; Buckthorn (Herb); Caffeine; Saturated fat;

Food Look-up Table for Ulcers

Food Item or Other	Suitability for Ulcers	Remarks (if any)
1-2 alcoholic drinks/day	Consume less	
2+ alcoholic drinks/day	Consume much less	
80+ proof distilled alc. bev.	Consume much less	
Abalone	Helpful	
Abiyuch	More helpful	
Acerola	More helpful	
Acorns	Neutral/OK	
After-dinner mints	Consume less	
Alcohol	Consume much less	
Alfalfa sprouts	Helpful	
Almonds	Helpful	
Amaranth	More helpful	
Amaranth leaves	Most helpful	
Anchovy	Helpful	
Antacids	More helpful	To neutralize stomach acid and reduce pain
Apple juice	More helpful	
Apples	More helpful	
Apples, dried	More helpful	
Applesauce	Neutral/OK	
Apricots	More helpful	
Apricots, dried	More helpful	
Arrowhead	More helpful	
Arrowroot	More helpful	
Artichoke	More helpful	
Artichoke, Jerusalem	More helpful	
Arugula	Most helpful	
Asparagus	Most helpful	
Aspirin	Avoid	also other NSAID drugs, e.g., ibuprofen, naproxen
Avocado	More helpful	
Bacon	Consume less	
Bagels	Neutral/OK	
Balsam pear	More helpful	
Balsam pear leafy tips	Most helpful	
Banana	More helpful	
Banana, dried	More helpful	
Barley	More helpful	
Basil (fresh)	Helpful	
Bass, freshwater	Neutral/OK	
Bass, Seabass	Neutral/OK	
Bass, striped	Neutral/OK	
Beans, adzuki	Helpful	
Beans, baked	Helpful	
Beans, black	Helpful	
Beans, black-eyed peas	Helpful	
Beans, fava	Helpful	
Beans, hyacinth	Helpful	
Beans, kidney	Helpful	
Beans, lima	Neutral/OK	
Beans, moth beans	Helpful	

Food Item or Other	Suitability for Ulcers Remarks (if any)
Beans, mung	Helpful
Beans, navy	Helpful
Beans, pinto	Helpful
Beans, winged	Helpful
Beans, yardlong	Helpful
Beans, yellow & white	Helpful
Bear meat	Helpful
Beaver meat	Neutral/OK
Beechnuts	Neutral/OK
Beef brain	Neutral/OK
Beef chuck/brisket	Neutral/OK
Beef filet mignon	Helpful
Beef heart	Neutral/OK
Beef jerky sticks	Neutral/OK
Beef kidneys	Neutral/OK
Beef liver	Helpful
Beef rib eye	Helpful
Beef ribs	Consume less
Beef round steak	Helpful
Beef shank	Neutral/OK
Beef spleen	Neutral/OK
Beef tenderloin/T-bone/portrhse	Neutral/OK
Beef tongue	Consume less
Beef top sirloin	Helpful
Beef, cured breakfast strips	Consume less
Beef, cured dried	Helpful
Beef, ground	Helpful
Beer	Consume less
Beerwurst beer salami	Consume less
Beet greens	Most helpful
Beets	More helpful
Bell peppers, green	More helpful
Bell peppers, red	More helpful
Biofeedback	Helpful
Biscuits	Consume less
Bison/buffalo meat	Neutral/OK
Blackberries	More helpful
Blueberries and Bilberries	More helpful
Bluefish	Neutral/OK
Boar meat	Neutral/OK
Bok choy	More helpful
Bologna, various	Consume less
Borage	More helpful
Boysenberries	More helpful
Brazil nuts	Neutral/OK
Bread sticks	Neutral/OK
Bread, banana	Neutral/OK
Bread, cornbread	Neutral/OK
Bread, Italian	Neutral/OK
Bread, oat bran	Neutral/OK
Bread, oat bran, rolls	Neutral/OK

Food Item or Other	Suitability for Ulcers	Remarks (if any)
Bread, pumpernickel	Helpful	
Bread, wheat germ	More helpful	
Bread, white	Consume less	
Bread, whole-wheat	More helpful	
Breadfruit	More helpful	
Breadfruit seeds	Helpful	
Broccoli	More helpful	sprouts in particular
Broccoli, Chinese	Most helpful	
Brussels sprouts	More helpful	
Buckthorn (Herb)	Consume much less	
Buckwheat	Most helpful	
Bulgur	More helpful	
Burbot	Neutral/OK	
Butter (salted)	Consume much less	
Butter (unsalted)	Consume much less	
Butterfish	Neutral/OK	
Butternuts	Helpful	
Cabbage, green	Most helpful	especially in juice form
Cabbage, red	Most helpful	especially in juice form
Cabbage, savoy	Most helpful	
Caffeine	Consume much less	
Cake, angel food	Consume less	
Cake, Boston cream pie	Consume less	
Cake, chocolate	Consume less	
Cake, gingerbread	Consume less	
Cake, pound	Consume much less	
Cake, shortcake	Consume less	
Cake, sponge	Consume less	
Cake, yellow	Consume less	
Calamari	Neutral/OK	
Candies, caramels	Neutral/OK	
Candies, carob	Consume less	
Candies, halvah	Helpful	
Candies, hard	Neutral/OK	
Candies, marshmallows	Neutral/OK	
Candies, peanut bar	Helpful	
Candies, peanut brittle	Neutral/OK	
Candies, sesame crunch	Helpful	
Candies, sweet chocolate	Avoid	
Cantaloupe	More helpful	
Capers	Neutral/OK	
Cardamom	Helpful	
Caribou meat	Helpful	
Carp	Neutral/OK	
Carrots	More helpful	
Cashew nuts	Helpful	
Catfish	Neutral/OK	
Cauliflower	More helpful	
Caviar	Consume less	
Cayenne (red) pepper	Helpful	
Celery	More helpful	

Food Item or Other	Suitability for Ulcers	Remarks (if any)
Celtuce	More helpful	
Cereal, bran flakes	Helpful	
Cereal, corn flakes	Neutral/OK	
Cereal, cream of wheat	Consume less	
Cereal, granola	Helpful	
Cereal, rice crisps	Consume less	
Cereal, shredded wheat	Helpful	
Cereal, wheat germ	More helpful	
Cereal, whole-wheat	More helpful	
Cheese fondue	Neutral/OK	
Cheese spread	Consume much less	
Cheese, American	Consume much less	
Cheese, blue	Consume much less	
Cheese, Brie	Consume much less	
Cheese, camembert	Consume much less	
Cheese, cheddar	Consume much less	
Cheese, Colby	Consume much less	
Cheese, cottage	Consume less	
Cheese, cream	Consume much less	
Cheese, edam	Consume much less	
Cheese, feta	Consume much less	
Cheese, Fontina	Consume much less	
Cheese, Gjetost	Consume much less	
Cheese, goat	Consume much less	
Cheese, gouda	Consume much less	
Cheese, gruyere	Consume much less	
Cheese, limburger	Consume much less	
Cheese, mozzarella	Consume much less	
Cheese, parmesan	Consume much less	
Cheese, pimento	Consume much less	
Cheese, port de Salut	Consume much less	
Cheese, ricotta	Consume much less	
Cheese, Romano	Consume much less	
Cheese, Roquefort	Consume much less	
Cheese, Swiss	Consume much less	
Cheeseburger	Neutral/OK	
Cheesecake	Consume less	
Cherries	More helpful	
Chervil	Neutral/OK	
Chestnuts	Helpful	
Chewing gum	Neutral/OK	
Chicken breast (no skin)	Neutral/OK	
Chicken dark meat	Neutral/OK	
Chicken giblets	Helpful	
Chicken heart	Helpful	
Chicken liver	Helpful	
Chicken Nuggets	Consume less	
Chicken skin	Consume less	
Chicken wings	Consume less	
Chickpeas	Helpful	
Chicory greens	Most helpful	

Food Item or Other	Suitability for Ulcers	Remarks (if any)
Chives	Neutral/OK	
Chocolate	Consume less	Avoid only if it bothers you
Chocolate mousse	Consume much less	
Chocolate, dark	Avoid	
Chorizo	Consume less	
Chrysanthemum (Garland)	Most helpful	
Chrysanthemum Leaves	More helpful	
Cinnamon	Helpful	stomach ulcer in particular
Cisco	Neutral/OK	
Cisco (smoked)	Neutral/OK	
Clams	Helpful	
Cloves	Helpful	
Cocoa	Consume much less	
Coconut	Consume less	
Coconut meat (dried)	Neutral/OK	
Coconut milk	Consume less	
Cod	Neutral/OK	
Coffee	Consume much less	
Coffee liqueur	Avoid	
Coffeecake	Consume less	
Cole slaw	Helpful	
Collards	Most helpful	
Consult your doctor	Most helpful; test for H. Pylori bacteria & eliminate with antibiotics	
Cookies, animal crackers	Consume less	
Cookies, brownies	Consume less	
Cookies, butter	Consume much less	
Cookies, chocolate chip	Consume much less	
Cookies, gingersnaps	Consume less	
Cookies, lady fingers	Consume less	
Cookies, molasses	Consume less	
Cookies, oatmeal	Consume less	
Cookies, peanut butter	Consume less	
Cookies, shortbread	Consume less	
Cookies, sugar	Consume less	
Cookies, vanilla wafers	Consume less	
Coriander/Cilantro	Helpful	
Corn	More helpful	
Corn bran	Most helpful	
Corn cakes	Neutral/OK	
Corned beef	Helpful	
Cornmeal, whole-grain	More helpful	
Cornnuts	Helpful	
Cottonseed meal	Helpful	
Couscous	Neutral/OK	
Cowberries	More helpful	
Cowpeas leafy tips	More helpful	
Crab, Alaskan King	Helpful	
Crab, blue	Helpful	
Crab, Dungeness	Helpful	
Crackers, matzo	Neutral/OK	
Crackers, melba toasts	Neutral/OK	

Food Item or Other	Suitability for Ulcers	Remarks (if any)
Crackers, milk	Consume less	
Crackers, saltines	Consume less	
Crackers, wheat	Neutral/OK	
Crackers, whole-wheat	More helpful	
Cranberries	More helpful	
Cranberry juice	More helpful	
Crayfish	Helpful	
Cream	Consume much less	
Cream puffs	Consume less	
Cream, whipped	Consume much less	
Crème de menthe	Consume much less	
Croaker	Consume less	
Croissant	Consume much less	
Croutons	Helpful	
Cucumbers with peel	More helpful	
Cured meats	Neutral/OK	
Currants (dried)	More helpful	
Currants (raw)	More helpful	
Cusk	Neutral/OK	
Cuttlefish	Helpful	
Dairy Products	Consume less	determine if this food allergen is a cause
Dandelion Greens	Most helpful	
Danish pastry	Consume less	
Dates	More helpful	
Dessert toppings	Consume less	
Detoxification	Helpful	3-day juice fast to alkalinize digestive tract
Dill weed	Neutral/OK	
Dolphinfish (Mahi-Mahi)	Neutral/OK	
Donuts	Consume less	
Drum	Neutral/OK	
Duck (no skin)	Neutral/OK	
Durian	More helpful	
Durum wheat	Most helpful	
Eat smaller, more frequent meals	Helpful	
Éclairs	Consume less	
Eel	Neutral/OK	
Egg (raw)	Neutral/OK	
Egg rolls (veg)	Neutral/OK	
Egg substitute	Neutral/OK	
Egg white	Neutral/OK	
Egg yolk	Consume less	
Egg, boiled & poached	Neutral/OK	
Egg, duck & goose	Neutral/OK	
Eggnog	Consume less	
Eggplant	More helpful	
Elderberries	More helpful	
Elimination diet	More helpful; to determine problem foods, e.g., milk, dairy, tea, chocolate, etc.	
Endive	Most helpful	
English muffins	Neutral/OK	
English muffins, whole-wheat	More helpful	
Epazote	More helpful	

Food Item or Other	Suitability for Ulcers	Remarks (if any)
Falafel	Neutral/OK	
Fasting (for a specific period)	Avoid	
Fat, beef/lamb/pork	Consume less	
Fat, chicken	Consume less	
Fat, goose/duck	Consume less	
Fat, saturated	Consume less	as part of a healthy diet
Fat, turkey	Consume less	
Fennel	More helpful	
Fennel seeds	Neutral/OK	
Fenugreek seeds	Neutral/OK	
Fiber	Helpful	soluble fiber in particular
Fiddlehead ferns	More helpful	
Figs	More helpful	
Figs, dried	More helpful	
Fish oil, cod liver	Consume less	
Fish oil, herring	Consume less	
Fish oil, menhaden	Consume less	
Fish oil, salmon	Consume less	
Fish oil, sardine	Consume less	
Fish roe	Helpful	
Flatfish (flounder & sole)	Neutral/OK	
Foie gras or liver pate	Consume less	
Food allergens	Consume much less	Determine if food allergy is a cause
Food prep -- fried or battered	Consume less	
Food prep -- spicy	Consume less	Is not a cause but could worsen symptoms
Frankfurter, beef and pork	Consume much less	
Frankfurter, chicken & turkey	Consume less	
French fries	Neutral/OK	
French toast	Consume less	
Frostings	Neutral/OK	
Frozen yogurt	Consume less	
Fruit leather/rolls	Consume less	
Fruit punch	Neutral/OK	
Fungi cloud ears	Most helpful	
Garden cress	Most helpful	
Garlic	More helpful	
German chamomile	Helpful	
Ginger	Neutral/OK	
Ginger ale	Neutral/OK	
Ginkgo nuts	Helpful	
Goji berry	More helpful	
Goose	Neutral/OK	
Gooseberries	More helpful	
Granola bars	Neutral/OK	
Grape juice	More helpful	
Grape leaves	Most helpful	
Grapefruit	Consume less	
Grapefruit juice	Consume less	
Grapes	More helpful	
Gravies (canned)	Neutral/OK	
Green beans	More helpful	

Food Item or Other	Suitability for Ulcers	Remarks (if any)
Green onions (scallions)	Most helpful	
Grouper	Neutral/OK	
Guarana	Consume less	
Guava	More helpful	
Guinea hen	Neutral/OK	
Haddock	Neutral/OK	
Halibut	Neutral/OK	
Hamburger	Neutral/OK	
Hash brown potatoes	Consume less	
Hazelnuts or Filberts	Helpful	
Hearts of palm	More helpful	
Herring	Neutral/OK	
Hickory nuts	Helpful	
Honey	More helpful	manuka honey for stomach ulcer in particular
Honeydew melon	More helpful	
Horseradish	Consume less	
Hot chocolate	Avoid	
Hot dog	Consume less	
Hummus	Neutral/OK	
Hush puppies	Neutral/OK	
Ice cream cones	Neutral/OK	
Ice cream, chocolate	Avoid	
Ice cream, vanilla	Consume less	
Irish Moss	Helpful	taken in specially prepared commercial form
Jams & Preserves	Neutral/OK	
Jellies	Neutral/OK	
Jujube (fruit)	More helpful	
Kale	Most helpful	
Kelp	Most helpful	
Ketchup	Consume less	
Kiwi fruit	Most helpful	
Kohlrabi	More helpful	
Kola (cola)	Consume less	
Kumquats	More helpful	
Lamb brain	Neutral/OK	
Lamb heart	Helpful	
Lamb kidneys	Helpful	
Lamb leg	Helpful	
Lamb liver	Helpful	
Lamb loin	Consume less	
Lamb ribs	Consume less	
Lamb shoulder	Neutral/OK	
Lamb spleen	Helpful	
Lamb tongue	Consume less	
Lamb, ground	Neutral/OK	
Lambsquarters	Helpful	
Lard	Consume less	
Leeks	More helpful	
Lemon	Consume less	
Lemonade	Neutral/OK	
Lentils	Helpful	

Food Item or Other	Suitability for Ulcers	Remarks (if any)
Lettuce, cos or Romaine	Most helpful	
Lettuce, head	More helpful	
Lettuce, loose leaf	Most helpful	
Licorice	More helpful	use in paste form
Lime	Consume less	
Ling	Neutral/OK	
Lingcod	Neutral/OK	
Litchi	More helpful	
Litchi, dried	More helpful	
Lobster	Helpful	
Lobster, spiny	Helpful	
Loganberry	More helpful	
Longans	More helpful	
Longans, dried	More helpful	
Lotus root	More helpful	
Luncheon meat, beef & pork	Consume much less	
Luncheon meat, cured beef	Consume less	
Lupin	Helpful	
Macadamia nuts	Consume less	
Macaroni	Consume less	
Mace	Neutral/OK	
Mackerel	Consume less	
Mackerel, king	Neutral/OK	
Malted drinks (nonalcoholic)	Consume less	
Mango	More helpful	
Margarine (salted)	Helpful	
Margarine (unsalted)	Helpful	
Margarine-like spreads	Neutral/OK	
Marjoram	Neutral/OK	
Marlin	Neutral/OK	
Mate	Consume less	
Mayonnaise	Helpful	
Milk	Consume much less	determine if milk allergy is a cause
Milk shakes	Consume less	
Milk, 2% fat	Consume less	
Milk, chocolate	Avoid	
Milk, low fat (1%)	Consume less	
Milk, Skim milk	Consume much less	
Milk, Whole milk	Consume less	
Milkfish	Neutral/OK	
Millet	More helpful	
Mints	Neutral/OK	
Miso	Helpful	
Molasses	Neutral/OK	
Molasses, blackstrap	Neutral/OK	
Monkfish	Neutral/OK	
Muffins, blueberry	Neutral/OK	
Muffins, corn	Neutral/OK	
Muffins, oat bran	Helpful	
Muffins, wheat bran	More helpful	
Mulberries	More helpful	

Food Item or Other	Suitability for Ulcers	Remarks (if any)
Mullet	Neutral/OK	
Mushrooms, Jew's ear	More helpful	
Mushrooms, portabella	More helpful	
Mushrooms, shitake	Most helpful	
Mussels	Helpful	
Mustard	Neutral/OK	
Mustard greens	Most helpful	
Mustard seed	Consume less	Avoid only if it bothers you
Mustard spinach	More helpful	
Nachos	Consume less	
Natal Plum (Carissa)	More helpful	
Natto	Helpful	
Nectarine	More helpful	
Non-dairy creamers	Consume less	
Noodles, Chinese chow Mein	Helpful	
Noodles, egg	Neutral/OK	
Noodles, Japanese	Neutral/OK	
Noodles, rice	Neutral/OK	
Nopal	More helpful	
Nutmeg	Consume less	Avoid only if it bothers you
Oat bran	Helpful	
Oatmeal (cereal)	More helpful	
Oats	Helpful	
Octopus	Helpful	
Oil, almonds	Neutral/OK	
Oil, apricot kernel	Neutral/OK	
Oil, avocado	Consume less	
Oil, Babassu	Consume less	
Oil, canola	Helpful	
Oil, Cocoa Butter	Consume less	
Oil, coconut	Consume less	
Oil, corn	Consume less	
Oil, cottonseed	Consume less	
Oil, Cupu Assu	Consume less	
Oil, flaxseed	Consume less	
Oil, grape seeds	Neutral/OK	
Oil, hazelnut	Neutral/OK	
Oil, hydrogenated vegetable	Consume less	
Oil, mustard	Consume less	
Oil, oat	Consume less	
Oil, olive	Helpful	
Oil, palm	Consume less	
Oil, peanut	Consume less	
Oil, poppy seed	Consume less	
Oil, rice bran	Consume less	
Oil, safflower	Neutral/OK	
Oil, sesame	Consume less	
Oil, Shea nut	Consume less	
Oil, soybean	Helpful	
Oil, sunflower	Consume less	
Oil, tea seed	Consume less	

Food Item or Other	Suitability for Ulcers	Remarks (if any)
Oil, tomato seeds	Consume less	
Oil, Ucuhuba Butter	Consume less	
Oil, walnut	Consume less	
Oil, wheat germ	Helpful	
Okra	More helpful	
Olives	More helpful	
Onion rings	Neutral/OK	
Onions	More helpful	
Orange juice	Consume less	
Orange roughy	Neutral/OK	
Oranges	Consume less	
Oregano	Helpful	
Oysters	Helpful	
Pancakes	Neutral/OK	
Pancreas (lamb, beef, veal)	Helpful	
Papaya	More helpful	
Parsley	Helpful	
Parsnips	More helpful	
Passion fruit	More helpful	
Pasta	Neutral/OK	
Pastrami, cured beef	Neutral/OK	
Pastrami, turkey	Consume less	
Peaches	More helpful	
Peaches, dried	More helpful	
Peanut butter	Neutral/OK	
Peanuts	Helpful	
Pears	More helpful	
Pears, dried	Most helpful	
Peas, green	Helpful	
Peas, split	More helpful	
Peas, sugar or snap	Helpful	
Pecans	Helpful	
Pepper (black or white)	Consume less	Avoid only if it bothers you
Pepper, banana	More helpful	
Peppermint	Helpful	
Pepperoni	Consume much less	
Peppers, ancho	Most helpful	
Peppers, hot chili	More helpful	
Peppers, hot chili, red	More helpful	
Peppers, jalapeno	More helpful	
Peppers, pasilla	Most helpful	
Peppers, pimento	More helpful	
Perch	Neutral/OK	
Persimmons	More helpful	
Pheasant	Neutral/OK	
Pheasant breast	Neutral/OK	
Pickle (cucumber)	Helpful	
Pickle relish	Neutral/OK	
Pickle, sweet	Helpful	
Pie crust	Consume less	
Pie, apple	Consume less	

Food Item or Other	Suitability for Ulcers Remarks (if any)
Pie, coconut cream	Consume less
Pie, fried pies (fruit)	Neutral/OK
Pie, lemon meringue	Neutral/OK
Pie, pecan	Neutral/OK
Pie, pumpkin	Neutral/OK
Pie, vanilla cream	Consume less
Pigeon peas	Most helpful
Pike, northern	Neutral/OK
Pike, walleye	Neutral/OK
Pili nuts	Consume less
Piña colada	Consume much less
Pine nuts	More helpful
Pineapple	More helpful
Pineapple juice	More helpful
Pistachio nuts	Helpful
Pitanga	More helpful
Pizza	Consume less
Plantains	More helpful
Plum	More helpful
Pokeberry shoots	Most helpful
Pollock	Neutral/OK
Pomegranate	More helpful
Pomegranate juice	More helpful
Pompano fish	Consume less
Popcorn, air popped	Most helpful
Popcorn, oil popped	More helpful
Poppy seed	Helpful
Pork back ribs	Consume less
Pork breakfast strips	Consume less
Pork cured/ham	Neutral/OK
Pork headcheese	Neutral/OK
Pork heart	Neutral/OK
Pork kidneys	Helpful
Pork leg/ham	Consume less
Pork liver	Helpful
Pork liver cheese	Consume less
Pork loin/sirloin	Neutral/OK
Pork lungs	Neutral/OK
Pork ribs	Consume less
Pork shldr	Neutral/OK
Pork skins	Consume less
Pork spare ribs	Consume less
Pork spleen	Helpful
Potato	More helpful
Potato chips/fried snacks	Helpful
Potato pancakes	Neutral/OK
Potato sticks	Consume less
Potatoes w/skin	More helpful
Pout	Neutral/OK
Prescription drugs	Avoid; NSAID (Nonsteroidal anti-inflammatory) and NSAID containing drugs
Pretzels	Neutral/OK

Food Item or Other	Suitability for Ulcers	Remarks (if any)
Prune juice	More helpful	
Prunes (dried)	Most helpful	
Pudding	Consume less	
Puff pastry	Consume less	
Pumelo (Shaddock)	Consume less	
Pumpkin	More helpful	
Pumpkin flowers	More helpful	
Pumpkinseed sunfish	Neutral/OK	
Purslane	More helpful	
Quail	Neutral/OK	
Quail breast	Neutral/OK	
Quince	More helpful	
Quinoa seed	More helpful	
Rabbit meat	Neutral/OK	
Radishes	More helpful	
Raisins	More helpful	
Raspberries	More helpful	
Raspberries, black	More helpful	
Rhubarb	More helpful	
Rice bran	More helpful	
Rice cakes (Brown rice based)	Helpful	
Rice, brown	More helpful	
Rice, white	Neutral/OK	
Rice, wild	More helpful	
Rockfish	Neutral/OK	
Rolls, dinner, Kaiser	Consume less	
Rolls, dinner, whole-wheat	Helpful	
Rolls, French	Consume less	
Rolls, hamburger & hot dog	Consume less	
Rosemary (fresh)	Helpful	
Rowal	More helpful	
Rutabaga	More helpful	
Rye	Most helpful	
Sablefish	Consume less	
Saffron	Neutral/OK	
Sage	Helpful	
Salad dressing, blue/Roquefort	Neutral/OK	
Salad dressing, French	Helpful	
Salad dressing, Italian	Neutral/OK	
Salami, various	Consume less	
Salmon (smoked, Lox)	Neutral/OK	
Salmon, pink	Neutral/OK	
Salt, table	Neutral/OK	
Sardines	Helpful	
Sauce, barbecue	Consume less	
Sauce, cheese	Consume less	
Sauce, fish	Consume less	
Sauce, Hoisin	Consume less	
Sauce, oyster	Consume less	
Sauce, pepper or hot	Consume less	
Sauce, Sofrito	Consume less	

Food Item or Other	Suitability for Ulcers	Remarks (if any)
Sauce, tabasco	Consume less	
Sauce, teriyaki	Helpful	
Sauerkraut	Helpful	
Sausage, blood	Consume much less	
Sausage, liver	Consume less	
Sausage, meatless	Consume less	
Sausage, various	Consume less	
Scallops	Neutral/OK	
Scup	Neutral/OK	
Seatrout	Neutral/OK	
Seeds, breadnut tree	Helpful	
Seeds, chia	More helpful	
Seeds, cottonseed	Helpful	
Seeds, flaxseed	More helpful	
Seeds, pumpkin & squash	Helpful	
Seeds, safflower	Helpful	
Seeds, sesame	Helpful	
Seeds, sunflower	Helpful	
Seeds, watermelon	Helpful	
Semolina	Neutral/OK	
Sesbania Flower	More helpful	
Shad	Neutral/OK	
Shallots	More helpful	
Shark	Neutral/OK	
Sheepshead	Neutral/OK	
Sherbet	Neutral/OK	
Shrimp	Helpful	
Shrimp, breaded	Neutral/OK	
Slippery Elm	Most helpful	stomach ulcer in particular
Smelt	Neutral/OK	
Smoking, tobacco	Consume much less	
Snail	Helpful	
Snapper	Neutral/OK	
Soft (carbonated) drinks	Consume less	
Sorghum	More helpful	
Soup, beef broth	Neutral/OK	
Soup, beef stock	Neutral/OK	
Soup, chicken broth	Neutral/OK	
Soup, chicken noodle	Neutral/OK	
Soup, chicken stock	Neutral/OK	
Soup, veg/beef	Neutral/OK	
Sour cream	Consume much less	
Soy milk	More helpful	
Soy sauce	Helpful	
Soybean seeds	More helpful	
Soybeans (green)	Helpful	
Spaghetti	Neutral/OK	
Spaghetti, spinach	Neutral/OK	
Spaghetti, whole-wheat	More helpful	
Spearmint (fresh)	Helpful	
Spelt (cooked)	More helpful	

Food Item or Other	Suitability for Ulcers	Remarks (if any)
Spinach	Most helpful	
Sports drinks	Neutral/OK	
Spot	Neutral/OK	
Squab (pigeon)	Consume less	
Squash, winter	More helpful	
Squash, yellow	More helpful	
Strawberries	More helpful	
Stress	Consume much less;	can worsen your symptoms
Sturgeon	Neutral/OK	
Succotash	Neutral/OK	
Sucker	Neutral/OK	
Sugar, brown	Neutral/OK	
Sugar, maple	Helpful	
Sugar, table (white or powder)	Consume less	
Surimi	Neutral/OK	
Sweet potatoes	More helpful	
Sweet potatoes leaves	Most helpful	
Sweet rolls	Consume less	
Swiss chard	Most helpful	
Swordfish	Neutral/OK	
Syrup, chocolate	Consume much less	
Syrup, malt	Neutral/OK	
Syrup, maple	Neutral/OK	
Syrup, sorghum	Neutral/OK	
Syrup, table blends	Neutral/OK	
Taco shells	Neutral/OK	
Tamarind	More helpful	
Tangerines	Consume less	
Tapioca	Consume less	
Taro	More helpful	
Taro chips	Neutral/OK	
Taro leaves	Most helpful	
Taro, Tahitian	More helpful	
Tarragon (dried)	Neutral/OK	
Tea, green	Consume less	
Tea, herbal	Neutral/OK	
Tea, plain	Consume less	Avoid if it bothers you
Tempeh	Helpful	
Thyme (fresh)	Helpful	
Tilapia	Neutral/OK	
Tilefish	Neutral/OK	
Toasted bread	Helpful	
Tofu	More helpful	
Tofu, fried	Helpful	
Tomato juice	More helpful	
Tomato paste	Helpful	
Tomatoes	More helpful	
Tomatoes, sun-dried	Most helpful	
Tonic water	Neutral/OK	
Tortilla chips	Helpful	
Tortillas (corn)	Helpful	

Food Item or Other	Suitability for Ulcers Remarks (if any)
Triticale	More helpful
Trout	Neutral/OK
Tuna, blue fin	Neutral/OK
Tuna, canned	Neutral/OK
Tuna, yellowfin	Neutral/OK
Turbot	Neutral/OK
Turkey breast	Neutral/OK
Turkey dark meat	Neutral/OK
Turkey giblets	Helpful
Turkey heart	Helpful
Turkey liver	Helpful
Turkey skins	Consume less
Turmeric	Neutral/OK
Turnip greens	Most helpful
Turnips	More helpful
Veal heart	Neutral/OK
Veal kidneys	Helpful
Veal liver	Helpful
Veal loin	Neutral/OK
Veal lungs	Neutral/OK
Veal shank	Helpful
Veal shoulder/leg/sirloin	Helpful
Veal spleen	Neutral/OK
Veal thymus	Neutral/OK
Veal tongue	Helpful
Vegetable shortening	Neutral/OK
Venison	Neutral/OK
Vine spinach (Basella)	More helpful
Vinegar	Neutral/OK
Vitamin E (Tocopherol)	Helpful
Vitamin K	Helpful
Waffles	Consume less
Walnuts	Neutral/OK
Walnuts, black	Helpful
Wasabi root	More helpful
Water	Helpful
Watercress	Most helpful
Watermelon	More helpful
Wheat	Neutral/OK
Wheat bran	More helpful
Wheat germ	More helpful
Whelk	Helpful
Whey (dried)	Consume less
Whiskey	Consume much less
White fish	Neutral/OK
White fish (smoked)	Neutral/OK
Whiting	Neutral/OK
Whole-wheat	Most helpful
Wine, red	Consume much less
Wine, white	Consume much less
Winged beans leaves	More helpful

Food Item or Other	Suitability for Ulcers Remarks (if any)
Wolffish	Neutral/OK
Yam	More helpful
Yellowtail	Neutral/OK
Yogurt	Helpful
Zinc	Helpful
Zucchini	More helpful

Anemia/Iron Deficiency & Ulcers

Hemoglobin is a type of protein that helps our red blood cells carry oxygen from our lungs to the rest of our body. Inability to produce adequate hemoglobin or lower than normal number of red blood cells in our blood result in Anemia which is a condition that refers to our blood's inability to carry enough oxygen to the rest of our body.

There are several types of Anemia. The type is normally associated with the root cause for Anemia. Loss of blood is the main cause for Anemia and can be due to factors such as heavy menstrual periods, bleeding from Ulcers or injuries, surgery, or cancer. Another cause for Anemia is inadequate production of red cells which can happen: if our diet is deficient in iron, Folic acid or Vitamin B-12; if our bone marrow does not produce enough red blood cells due to low level of the needed erythropoietin hormone; due to certain diseases (e.g., kidney or cancer) or certain medical treatments (such as for cancer or AIDS/HIV); and in case of pregnancy. The third cause is high rate of destruction of red blood cells which can happen due to an abnormal spleen (which is responsible for removing old red blood cells), or certain diseases and inherited conditions.

Women of childbearing age, pregnant women, and older adults are at a higher risk of developing Anemia.

Anemia is a common condition, and in most cases can be easily treated through diet.

The most likely cause of Anemia is iron deficiency, and thus the focus of this section. Our body needs iron to make hemoglobin.

Choose these for Ulcers & Anemia

Top 5 items to choose:

Green leafy vegetables; Dried fruits; Liver; Sun-dried tomatoes; Amaranth;

Food items and actions that could improve your health (within a food group, most helpful items are listed first):

Meat, Fish & Poultry

Liver; Chicken & turkey heart; Cuttlefish; Octopus; Clams; Whelk; Chicken giblets; Kidneys; Spleen; Chicken liver; Heart; Pork lungs; Mussels; Game meat; Veal thymus; Caviar; Turkey giblets; Venison; Pancreas (lamb, beef, veal); Oysters; Pork liver cheese; Veal lungs; Quail; Liver sausage; Abalone; Calamari; Anchovy; Rabbit meat; Duck (no skin); Fish roe; Beef jerky sticks; Dungeness crab; King mackerel; Trout; Lobster; Alaskan king crab; Quail breast; Snail; Crayfish; Blue crab; Meatless sausage; Squab (pigeon); Shad; Spot; Blue fin tuna; Boar meat; Spiny lobster; Drum; Lamb brain; Goose; Walleye; Pork headcheese; Bison/buffalo meat; Beef round steak; Sucker;

Eggs, Beans, Nuts and Seeds

Soybean seeds; Breadnut tree seeds; Split peas; Seeds: sesame, chia, pumpkin & squash, flaxseed; Sugar or snap peas; Seeds: safflower, watermelon; Soybeans (green); Cashew nuts; Pine nuts; Soy milk; Sunflower seeds; Fava beans; Cottonseed; Green peas; Winged beans; Pistachio nuts; Chestnuts; Almonds; Ginkgo nuts; Breadfruit seeds; Beechnuts; Hyacinth beans; Butternuts; Black walnuts; Coconut meat (dried); Pecans; Chickpeas; Lentils; Egg substitute; Duck & goose eggs; Peanuts; Acorns; Kidney beans; Hazelnuts or Filberts; Walnuts; Black-eyed peas; various beans; Alfalfa sprouts; Macadamia nuts; Hickory nuts; Cornnuts; Pili nuts; Lupin; Boiled & poached eggs;

Fruits & Juices

Dried fruits: Peaches, Longans, Goji berry, Litchi; Persimmons; Prunes (dried); Abiyuch; Kiwi fruit; Currants (dried); Guava; Raisins; Dried pears; Rowal; Dried Banana, Apricots; Elderberries; Currants (raw); Passion fruit; Litchi; Longans; Tamarind; Dried fruits; Olives; Kumquats; Acerola; Jujube (fruit); Papaya; Strawberries; Pineapple juice; Dates; Mulberries; Pineapple; Natal Plum (Carissa); Blackberries; Cantaloupe; Mango; Pomegranate; Avocado; Breadfruit; Boysenberries; Raspberries; Blueberries and Bilberries; Cranberries; Durian; Figs; Grapes; Pears; Pomegranate juice; Plantains; Gooseberries; Apple juice; Apples; Apricots; Cherries; Cranberry juice; Grape juice; Nectarine; Peaches; Plum; Prune juice; Watermelon; Loganberry; Cowberries; Pitanga; Banana; Honeydew melon; Quince; Lemon; Orange juice; Oranges; Pumelo (Shaddock);

Vegetables

Sun-dried tomatoes; Taro leaves; Ancho & Pasilla peppers; Balsam pear leafy tips; Kale; Fungi cloud ears; Pigeon peas; Beet greens; Turnip greens; Dandelion Greens; Mustard greens; Garden cress; Pokeberry shoots; Jalapeno peppers; Winged beans leaves; Amaranth leaves; Hot chili peppers; Grape leaves; Shitake mushrooms; Pimento peppers; Collards; Red cabbage (juice in particular); Watercress; Swiss chard; Mustard spinach; Borage; Broccoli (sprouts in particular); Lambsquarters; Bok choy; Tahitian taro; Balsam pear; Savoy cabbage; Kohlrabi; Banana peppers; Cowpeas leafy tips; Wasabi root; Chinese broccoli; Green bell peppers; Sesbania Flower; Green cabbage (juice in particular); Vine spinach (Basella); Red bell peppers; Chicory greens; Cauliflower; Kelp; Romaine & loose leaf lettuce; Sweet potatoes leaves; Brussels sprouts; Chrysanthemum (Garland); Green onions (scallions); Okra; Arugula; Purslane; Endive; Leeks; Lotus root; Garlic; Head lettuce; Jerusalem artichoke; Pumpkin flowers; Parsnips; Hearts of palm; Epazote; Asparagus; Rutabaga; Jew's ear mushrooms; Artichoke; Sweet potatoes; Chrysanthemum Leaves; Arrowroot; Fiddlehead ferns; Carrots; Radishes; Celery; Green beans; Celtuce; Yellow squash; Tomato juice; Zucchini; other vegetables;

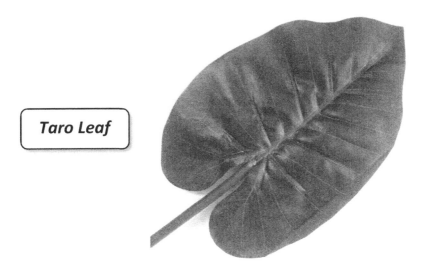

Taro Leaf

Breads, Grains, Cereals, Pasta

Amaranth; Wheat germ cereal; Rice bran; Wheat germ; Bran flakes; Rye; Buckwheat; Corn bran; Whole-wheat; Durum wheat; Sorghum; Whole-wheat cereal; Triticale; Whole-wheat crackers; Oats; Corn flakes; Rice crisps; Whole-wheat spaghetti; Oatmeal (cereal); Whole-wheat bread; Bread sticks; Spelt (cooked); Toasted bread; Whole-wheat English muffins; Chinese chow Mein noodles; Oat bran muffins; Wheat germ bread; Saltines; Wheat crackers; Pumpernickel bread; Wheat bran muffins; Corn muffins; Barley; Bulgur; Italian bread; Oat bran bread; Granola cereal; Whole-wheat dinner rolls; Shredded wheat cereal; Millet; Corn; Brown rice; Wild rice; Melba toasts crackers; Banana bread; Kaiser dinner rolls; Biscuits; Matzo crackers; French rolls; Oat bran; Wheat bran; White bread; Milk crackers; Cream of wheat; Granola bars;

Dairy Products, Fats & Oils

Wheat germ oil; Yogurt;

Desserts, Snacks, Beverages

Air popped popcorn; Ice cream cones; Pretzels; Halvah; Honey (Manuka honey for stomach ulcer in particular); Gingersnaps cookies; Molasses cookies; Molasses; Sesame crunch candies; Oil popped popcorn; Fruit leather/rolls; Potato sticks; Lady fingers cookies;

Herbs & Spices, Fast Foods, Prepared Foods

Parsley; Natto; Thyme (fresh); Rosemary (fresh); Peppermint; Spearmint (fresh); Tofu; Whole-grain cornmeal; Fried tofu; Cottonseed meal; Soy sauce; Dill weed; Basil (fresh); Croutons; Teriyaki sauce; Coriander/Cilantro; Tempeh; Tomato paste; Cole slaw; Corn salad; Cayenne (red) pepper; Foie gras or liver pate; Miso; Sorghum syrup; Cinnamon (stomach ulcer in particular); Potato pancakes; Falafel; Tarragon (dried); Hummus; Hush puppies; Hamburger; Sage; Mace; Succotash; Turmeric; Clam chowder; Maple & Malt syrups;

Alternative therapies & Miscellaneous

Consult your doctor (need to confirm the cause of Anemia & test for H. Pylori bacteria); Elimination diet (need to determine foods that cause problems for Ulcers, milk, dairy, tea, chocolate, etc.); Prepare food in cast-iron pot;

Key Nutrients & Herbal Medicines

Iron; Slippery Elm (for stomach ulcer in particular); Anise, anise seed (star anise in particular); Licorice (user in paste form); Vitamin C (Ascorbic acid);

Do not choose these for Ulcers & Anemia

Top 5 items to avoid:

Aspirin & Prescription drugs; Alcohol & Smoking;
Coffee; Fasting; Cheese;

Avoid or consume much less of the following (within a food group, most harmful items are listed first):

Meat, Fish & Poultry

Beef & pork luncheon meat; Beef and pork frankfurter; Sausage; Chorizo; Pepperoni;

Instead _Choose_: **Mackerel; Sardines; Butterfish; Ling; Pollock; Rockfish; Tilefish; Burbot; Cisco (smoked); Salmon (smoked, Lox); White fish (smoked); Ground beef; Tongue; Herring; Carp; Pumpkinseed sunfish; Turkey pastrami; Scallops; Seabass; Striped bass; Bluefish; Catfish; Cisco; Cod; Cusk; Dolphinfish (Mahi-Mahi); Flatfish (flounder & sole); Grouper; Haddock; Halibut; Lingcod; Milkfish; Monkfish; Mullet; Northern pike; Pink salmon; Scup; Seatrout; Shark; Sheepshead; Snapper; Sturgeon; Surimi; Tilapia; Canned tuna; Yellowfin tuna; Turbot; Whiting; Wolffish; Yellowtail; Turkey dark meat; Freshwater bass; Pout; White fish; Smelt; Shrimp; Pheasant breast; Guinea hen; Pheasant; Cured beef; Marlin; Orange roughy; Swordfish; Turkey breast; Eel; Perch; Croaker; Lamb leg; Corned beef; Beef filet mignon; Beef chuck/brisket; Sablefish;**

Eggs, Beans, Nuts and Seeds

Egg yolk; Brazil nuts;

Instead _Choose_: **Egg; Egg white; Coconut;**

Fruits & Juices

There are no fruits that can worsen your condition.

Instead _Choose_: **Rhubarb; Grapefruit juice; Lime; Grapefruit; Tangerines;**

Vegetables

There are no vegetables that can worsen your condition.

Breads, Grains, Cereals, Pasta

There are no items in this food group that would worsen your condition.

Instead _Choose_: **Cornbread; Rice cakes (Brown rice based); Hamburger & hot dog rolls; Tortillas (corn); Waffles; Semolina; Spinach spaghetti; Wheat; Bagels; Sweet rolls; Couscous; Blueberry muffins; various noodles; Pasta; White rice; Spaghetti;**

Dairy Products, Fats & Oils

Various cheese; Milk (determine if you are allergic to milk); Butter; Whipped cream; Chocolate milk; Oils: Babassu, corn, palm, peanut, poppy seed; various seeds/nuts/vegetable oils; Sour cream; Animal fats; Poultry fats; Lard; Hydrogenated vegetable oil; Margarine-like spreads; Margarine; Olive oil;

Instead _Choose_: Goat cheese; various fish oil; Non-dairy creamers; Canola oil; Flaxseed oil; Apricot kernel oil; Walnut oil;

Desserts, Snacks, Beverages

Coffee; Coffee liqueur; Red wine; 80+ proof distilled alcoholic beverages; Whiskey; Plain tea (avoid only if it bothers you); Crème de menthe; Chocolate ice cream; Hot chocolate; Piña colada; White wine; Sweet chocolate; Pound cake; Carob candies; Vanilla ice cream; Dessert toppings; Taro chips; Frozen yogurt; Milk shakes; Chocolate chip cookies; Beer;

Instead _Choose_: Animal crackers cookies; Potato chips/fried snacks; Sponge cake; Puff pastry; Tortilla chips; Oatmeal cookies; Gingerbread cake; Peanut butter cookies; Shortbread cookies; Water; Shortcake; Chocolate (avoid if it bothers you); Pancakes; Peanut bar; Pie crust; Pecan pie; Brownies; Caramel candies; Tapioca; Applesauce; Fruit punch; Ginger ale; Lemonade; Herbal tea; Tonic water;

Herbs & Spices, Fast Foods, Prepared Foods

Cheese sauce; Cocoa; Nachos; Table sugar (white or powder); Chocolate syrup; Nutmeg (avoid if it bothers you);

Instead _Choose_: Cheeseburger; Oregano; Fennel seeds; Sweet pickle; Sauerkraut; Egg rolls (veg); Mustard; Fish stock; Chervil; Poppy seed; Cardamom; Corn cakes; Cloves; Chives; Pickle (cucumber); Saffron; French toast; Mints; Sofrito sauce; Maple sugar; Capers; Taco shells;

Alternative therapies & Miscellaneous

Smoking, tobacco; Aspirin & other NSAID drugs; Fasting (for a specific period); Prescription drugs (NSAID and NSAID containing drugs); 2+ alcoholic drinks/day; Food allergens (determine if Ulcers is triggered by an allergy); Stress;

Key Nutrients & Herbal Medicines

Alcohol; Buckthorn (Herb); Caffeine;

Cancer Risk & Ulcers

Cells are the building block of every organ in our body. Cells reproduce or die at varying rates depending on the organ and our age. Sometimes we have abnormal cells that reproduce or divide at a faster rate than we need. This phenomenon results in a collection of unwanted cells called a tumor. If the cells in the tumor have the ability to infiltrate other tissues and organs in our body then this tumor is considered malignant, otherwise it is considered benign. Cancer is the condition that corresponds to the malignant tumors. Cancer refers to as many as 200 different diseases but they all have the out of control cell reproduction in common.

Cancers are named after the organ where a tumor first appears. Some cancers do not form a tumor such as cancer of blood. In medical jargon, if cancer affects soft tissues and organs such as breast or lung, they are categorized as Carcinomas. If cancer affects hard tissues such as bone or muscle, they are called Sarcomas. If cancer affects our lymphatic system (i.e., part of body's circulatory system which transports things such as plasma, fats, white cells from one place to another throughout our body), it is called Lymphoma. And finally if cancer affects tissues such as blood or bone marrow, it is known as Leukemia.

There has been significant progress in cancer research and treatment of cancer over the recent decades. We understand that gene mutations are the cause of cancer development. We also know of most of the causes for gene mutations that cause cancer, i.e., the carcinogens. In short, the research has led to identification of various risk factors that increase the possibility of developing cancer. The most common of which are: family history of cancer; age (growing older); exposure to Ultraviolet (UV) radiation (from sun, tanning booths, sunlamps); certain infections; hormones (e.g., estrogen); exposure to certain chemicals (e.g., radon gas, asbestos); alcohol; tobacco; poor diet; stress; obesity and lack of physical activity. Having several risk factors does NOT mean that one will get cancer. Conversely, absence of risk factors does not mean that one will not get cancer.

The suggestions and information presented in this book are primarily focused on <u>prevention</u> of various cancer types through avoidance of the known risk factors for the specific cancer type. When known, information about food items or actions that could shrink or slow down growth of tumors is included. It is important to note that, there is no definitive cure, treatment or preventive measure that is known and certain for any specific type of cancer at this time.

Few words on phytochemicals, antioxidants, free radicals ...

Phytochemicals are substances or compounds found in many plants. They are also known by other names among them antioxidants and flavonoids. While thousands of phytochemicals have been discovered, very few have been studied in detail. Some of the better known phytochemicals (antioxidants) are beta carotene, Vitamin C, folic acid and Vitamin E.

Various studies and many experts suggest that the risk of cancer can be significantly reduced by eating more fruits, vegetables, beans and whole grains that contain phytochemicals. There is some evidence that certain phytochemicals may prevent formation of tumors, or suppress cancer development. But there is no data that supports taking phytochemical supplements is as effective as consuming fruits, vegetables, beans and grains as part of a normal diet. Nor are supplements regulated by the FDA. Thus, taking phytochemicals in form of supplements is not recommended.

One group of these compounds, known as antioxidants, may protect our cells against free radicals. Free radicals are molecules produced by our body as it breaks down food or by exposure to things such as tobacco smoke or radiation. Free radicals can damage our cell's DNA and are linked to certain diseases including cancer. Antioxidants are thought to eliminate free radicals, and slow down oxidation, which is a natural process that leads to damage to the cells and tissue in our body.

Another group of these compounds is known as flavonoids. Some studies suggest that some of these compounds may protect against hormone-dependent cancers such as breast and prostate cancers. Another group of flavonoids act as antioxidants, and thus have protective and anti-cancer properties.

A third group of Phytochemicals, called Allyl Sulfides, may help our body get rid of harmful chemicals and strengthen our immune system.

Many of the dietary recommendations that you find in this chapter are based on the various known phytochemical content and their effect on various types of cancer.

Choose these for Ulcers & Cancer Risk

Top 5 items to choose:

Green leafy vegetables/Cabbage; Sun-dried tomatoes; Prunes/Dried Fruits; Mushrooms; Rye;

Food items and actions that could improve your health or reduce your risk (within a food group, the most helpful items are listed first):

Meat, Fish & Poultry

Fish roe; Turkey & chicken liver; Chicken & turkey giblets; Spiny lobster; Pink salmon; Pork liver; Dungeness crab; Oysters; Alaskan king crab; Blue crab; Herring; White fish; Ling; Seabass; Sturgeon; Pout; Smelt; Snail; Pompano fish; Octopus; Spot; Mussels; Trout; Eel; Mackerel; Pollock; Whiting; Wolffish; Crayfish; Sardines; Anchovy; Beef liver; Snapper; Scup; Blue fin tuna; Abalone; Yellowtail;

Eggs, Beans, Nuts and Seeds

Soy milk; Split peas; Fava beans; Soybeans (green); Green peas; Alfalfa sprouts; Breadnut tree seeds; Beans: black, navy, yellow & white; Chickpeas; Lentils; Hyacinth beans; Chia seeds; Adzuki beans; Black-eyed peas; Mung & pinto beans; Sugar or snap peas; Various beans; Flaxseed (take ground seeds with water); Sunflower seeds; Lupin; Ginkgo nuts; Hazelnuts or Filberts; Almonds; Soybean seeds; Peanuts; Breadfruit seeds; Walnuts; Chestnuts; Pine nuts; Safflower seeds; Coconut meat (dried); Beechnuts; Sesame seeds; Egg yolk; Pistachio nuts; Cottonseed; Brazil nuts;

Fruits & Juices (Five servings of fruits & Veg daily. Avoid non-organic. Wash fruits & vegetables well and peel their skin)

Prunes (dried); Dried pears; Kiwi fruit; Blackberries; Passion fruit; Dried peaches; Plantains; Dried banana; Dried apricots; Boysenberries; Currants (dried); Guava; Kumquats; Raspberries; Rhubarb; Rowal; Loganberry; Abiyuch; Tamarind; various berries; Cranberries; Currants (raw); Dried fruits; Apricots; Cantaloupe; Mango; Papaya; Peaches; Persimmons; Plum; Acerola; Cranberry juice; Watermelon; Blueberries and Bilberries; Pitanga; Breadfruit; Nectarine; Jujube (fruit); Litchi; Longans; Avocado; Raisins; Pomegranate; Dates; Durian; Natal Plum (Carissa); Pineapple juice; Pineapple; Apples; Grapes; Figs; Olives; Pears; Banana; Cherries; Quince; Apple juice; Pomegranate juice; Honeydew melon; Grape juice; Prune juice; Strawberries; Lemon; Grapefruit; Oranges;

Vegetables *(Five servings of fruits & Veg daily. Avoid non-organic. Wash fruits & vegetables well and peel their skin)*

Grape leaves; Shitake mushrooms; Sun-dried tomatoes; Pigeon peas; Sweet potatoes leaves; Green & red cabbage (juice in particular); Dandelion Greens; Beet greens; Chicory greens; Collards; Mustard greens; Taro leaves; Turnip greens; Chinese broccoli; Savoy cabbage; Chrysanthemum (Garland); Endive; Fungi cloud ears; Green onions (scallions); Ancho & pasilla peppers; Spinach; Swiss chard; Amaranth leaves; Arugula; Balsam pear leafy tips; Garden cress; Kale; Romaine & loose leaf lettuce; Pokeberry shoots; Watercress; Artichoke; Bok choy; Okra; Wasabi root; Kelp; Jalapeno peppers; Epazote; Green beans; Head lettuce; Cauliflower; Chrysanthemum Leaves; Kohlrabi; Mustard spinach; Banana peppers; Sweet potatoes; Winged beans leaves; Parsnips; Bell peppers; Borage; Celtuce; Cowpeas leafy tips; Hot chili peppers; Pimento peppers; Pumpkin; Pumpkin flowers; Purslane; Radishes; Rutabaga; Sesbania Flower; Winter squash; Tahitian taro; Vine spinach (Basella); Asparagus; Turnips; Taro; Arrowroot; Leeks; Tomato juice; Garlic (take raw or crushed but not heated immediately); Lambsquarters; Broccoli (sprouts in particular); Brussels sprouts; Lotus root; Yam; other vegetables;

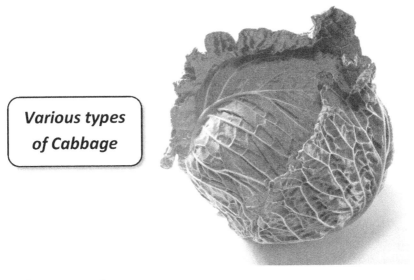

Various types of Cabbage

Breads, Grains, Cereals, Pasta

Rye; Corn bran; Buckwheat; Amaranth; Barley; Sorghum; Oats; Corn; Oatmeal (cereal); Rice bran; Wild rice; Bran flakes cereal; Millet; Brown rice; Oat bran; Rice cakes (Brown rice based); Tortillas (corn); Triticale;

Dairy Products, Fats & Oils

Yogurt; Cod Liver Fish Oil; Wheat Germ Oil; Fat-free or Low Fat products

Desserts, Snacks, Beverages

Air-popped Popcorn; Water (pure water, not tap water); Oil-popped popcorn; Green tea (do not brew or drink boiling hot); Pumpkin pie;

Herbs & Spices, Fast Foods, Prepared Foods

Tofu; Coriander/Cilantro; Parsley; Thyme (fresh); Whole-grain cornmeal; Peppermint; Spearmint (fresh); Tempeh; Egg rolls (veg); Minestrone soup; Cayenne (red) pepper; Dill weed; Vegetable soup; Basil (fresh); Corn salad; Fried tofu; Natto; Cole slaw; Rosemary (fresh); Maple sugar; Oregano; Sage; Tomato paste; Cinnamon (helps stomach ulcer in particular); Cottonseed meal; Mints; Croutons; Mace; Turmeric; Miso; Chives; Marjoram; Teriyaki sauce; Succotash; Cardamom; Veg/beef soup;

Alternative Therapies & Miscellaneous

Consult your doctor (ask for screening for cancer & test for H. Pylori bacteria); Antacids; Anti-inflammation diet; Detoxification (3-day juice fast to alkalinize digestive tract); Elimination diet (to determine which foods cause problems for your ulcer, e.g., milk, dairy, tea, chocolate, etc.); Exercise; Organically grown foods; Wild fish and free range animals (avoid animals raised on antibiotics or grain fed); Alkaline diet;

Key Nutrients & Herbal Medicines

Fiber (soluble fiber in particular); Slippery Elm (helps stomach ulcer in particular); Beta Carotene (do not take in supplement form); Bugleweed; Foxglove; Licorice (use in paste form); Zinc; Vitamin E (Tocopherol);

Do not choose these for Ulcers & Cancer Risk

Top 5 items to avoid:

Chocolate & Sweets; Cheese; Luncheon (processed) Meats; Butter; Smoking & Alcohol;

Avoid or consume much less of the following (within a food group, most harmful items are listed first):

Meat, Fish & Poultry

Blood sausage; Pepperoni; Frankfurters; Luncheon meats; Chorizo; various sausage; Pastrami; Salami; Pork skins; Bacon; Pork breakfast strips; Turkey skins; Bologna; Cured beef; Pork liver cheese; Beef tongue; Pork spare ribs; Beef jerky sticks; Beef ribs; Pork cured/ham; Pork ribs; Lamb tongue; Lamb ribs; Corned beef; Pork headcheese; Ground beef; Lamb loin; Pork; Salmon (smoked, Lox); Lamb; Beef; Cured meats; Meat (limit consumption of red meat; choose organic); Chicken skin; Organ meats; Rabbit meat; Venison; Veal loin; Bison/buffalo meat; White fish (smoked); Squab (pigeon); Veal; Boar meat; Orange roughy; Shark; Goose; Grouper; Sablefish; Croaker; King mackerel; Tilefish; Yellowfin tuna; Pheasant; Quail; Chicken dark meat;

Instead **choose**: Lingcod; Catfish; Mullet; Tilapia; Calamari; Shad; Clams; Cusk; Dolphinfish (Mahi-Mahi); Turbot; Turkey heart; Veal liver; Whelk; Lobster; Shrimp; Monkfish; Lamb liver; Freshwater bass; Sucker; Walleye; Surimi; Sheepshead; Cuttlefish; Pancreas (lamb, beef, veal); Flatfish (flounder & sole); Chicken heart; Carp; Rockfish; Halibut; Striped bass; Drum; Marlin; Caviar; Butterfish; Milkfish; Cod; Cisco; Chicken breast; Turkey dark meat; Seatrout; Burbot; Northern pike; Swordfish; Haddock;

Eggs, Beans, Nuts and Seeds

Coconut milk; Pili nuts; Pumpkin & squash seeds;

Instead **choose**: Acorns; Pecans; Egg; Black walnuts; Cornnuts; Egg substitute; Watermelon seeds; Egg white; Macadamia nuts; Coconut; Cashew nuts;

Fruits & Juices

Avoid sugared fruits juices or made from concentrate;

Breads, Grains, Cereals, Pasta

Danish pastry; Milk crackers; Croissant; Saltines crackers; Donuts; Sweet rolls; Wheat crackers; Granola bars; Hamburger & hot dog rolls; White bread; Wheat; Biscuits; French rolls; Kaiser dinner rolls; Matzo crackers; Cream of wheat; Melba toasts crackers; Rice crisps cereal; Banana bread; Bagels; Cornbread; Blueberry muffins;

Instead **choose**: Chinese chow Mein noodles; Wheat bran muffins; Oat bran muffins; Whole-wheat; Granola cereal; Couscous; Egg noodles; Spaghetti; Spinach spaghetti; Shredded wheat cereal; Durum wheat; Wheat germ cereal; Bulgur; Spelt (cooked); Whole-wheat bread; Whole-wheat English muffins; Whole-wheat cereal; Whole-wheat spaghetti; Whole-wheat dinner rolls; Wheat germ bread; Whole-wheat crackers;

Dairy Products, Fats & Oils

American cheese; Chocolate milk; Butter; Cheese: Romano, Parmesan, Roquefort; Cheese spread; various cheese; Milk (determine if you are allergic to milk); Vegetable shortening; Animal fat; Hydrogenated vegetable oil; Whipped cream; Poultry fat; Lard; Sesame oil; Oils: Cupu Assu, Shea nut, tea seed, Ucuhuba Butter; Cream; Dairy Products (determine if you are allergic to them); various seeds/nuts/vegetable oils; Sour cream; Margarine-like spreads; Corn oil;

Instead choose: Canola oil; Olive oil; various fish oil; Hazelnut oil; Safflower oil;

Desserts, Snacks, Beverages

Chocolate chip cookies; Chocolate ice cream; Sweet chocolate; various cakes; various cookies; Coffee liqueur; Puff pastry; Éclairs; Pudding; Cream puffs; Chocolate mousse; Dark chocolate; Hot chocolate; 80+ proof distilled alcoholic beverages.; Chocolate (avoid if it bothers you); Dessert toppings; Whiskey; Coffee; Pretzels; Cheesecake; Crème de menthe; Coffeecake; Coconut cream pie; Pie crust; Soft (carbonated) drinks; Vanilla ice cream; After-dinner mints; Fruit leather/rolls; various pies; Frozen yogurt; Piña colada; Candies; Pancakes; White wine; Tortilla chips; Peanut brittle candies; Marshmallows; Halvah; various candies; Ice cream cones; Beer; Taro chips; Lemonade; Chewing gum; Milk shakes; Molasses;

Instead choose: Red wine; Sesame crunch candies; Herbal tea; Blackstrap molasses; Honey; Plain tea;

Herbs & Spices, Fast Foods, Prepared Foods

Cheese sauce; Table sugar (white or powder); Nachos; Hot dog; Pizza; Barbecue sauce; Oyster sauce; Chicken Nuggets; various sauces; Breaded shrimp; Blue/Roquefort salad dressing; Hush puppies; Italian salad dressing; Cheeseburger; French salad dressing; Ketchup; Tapioca; Macaroni; Tabasco sauce; Chocolate syrup; Onion rings; Hamburger; Beef broth; Mayonnaise; Foie gras or liver pate; Malt syrup; Table salt; Taco shells; Syrup (table blends); Mustard seed (avoid only if bothers you); Beef stock; Pickle relish; Capers; Gravies (canned);

Instead choose: Cloves; Sauerkraut; Chervil; French fries; Poppy seed; Tarragon (dried); Ginger; Fennel seeds; Tomato soup; Brown sugar; Potato pancakes; Soy sauce; Chicken stock; Chicken broth; Fish stock; Sweet pickle; Saffron; Pepper (black & white); Nutmeg (avoid if it bothers you); Vinegar; Mustard; Horseradish; Cheese fondue; Falafel;

Alternative Therapies & Miscellaneous

Smoking, tobacco; Alcoholic drinks; Stress; Processed or Refined foods; Prescription drugs (NSAID and NSAID containing drugs); Fasting (for a specific period); Pesticide-loaded crops; Air pollutants; Aspirin (& other NSAID drugs such as ibuprofen and naproxen); Food additives Nitrates/Nitrites; Food allergens (determine if any allergy causes ulcer problems); Fried or battered foods; Smoked food/fish; Harsh chemicals & fumes; Non-organic foods; Radiation (from X-rays, television, microwave, computer, cell phones); Corn sweetener;

Key Nutrients & Herbal Medicines

Alcohol; Caffeine; Betel Nut; Buckthorn (Herb); Mercury (avoid heavy metal loaded fish); Trans fatty acids; Saturated fat; Guarana; Kola (cola); Mate;

Depression & Ulcers

Depression is a serious chronic illness. It is not just a temporary feeling of being down. It is a disorder of the brain. It can interfere with your normal life and lead to various physical and emotional problems. It affects men, women and elderly in different ways.

The exact cause of depression is unknown. But several factors can lead to depression: loss of a loved one, stressful situations such as a difficult relationship or financial problems, family history of depression (genetic factors), differences in brain chemistry, changes in body hormones, and traumatic events during one's childhood.

You are more likely to get depression if you are between 15 and 30 years old, you are a woman, it is winter time, or it is just after you gave birth to a baby.

Choose these for Ulcers & Depression

Top 5 items to choose:

Whole Grains; Soymilk/Soybeans; Peas;
Sun-dried tomatoes; Seeds;

Food items and actions that could improve your health (within a food group, most helpful items are listed first):

Meat, Fish & Poultry

Liver; Anchovy; Mussels; Chicken & turkey giblets; Fish roe; Chicken & turkey heart; Pork kidneys; Marlin; Swordfish; White fish; Cuttlefish; Spiny lobster; Bluefish; Ling; King mackerel; Milkfish; Pink salmon; Spot; Tilefish; Trout; Blue fin tuna; Sardines; Herring; Striped bass; Alaskan king crab; Kidneys; Seabass; Octopus; Shad; Shark; Wolffish; Smelt; Caviar; Whelk; Mackerel; Pollock; Calamari; Dungeness crab; Drum; Yellowtail; Clams; Scup; Heart; Meatless sausage; Yellowfin tuna; Pout; Cisco (smoked); Monkfish; Walleye; Pompano fish; Pork loin/sirloin; Pork cured/ham; Sucker; Carp; Whiting; Freshwater bass; Animal brain; Venison; Veal shank; Snapper; Sablefish; Chicken breast (no skin); Quail; Pancreas (lamb, beef, veal); Beef filet mignon; Burbot; Mullet; Oysters; Surimi; Cured beef; Abalone; Shrimp; Blue crab; Beef round steak; Spleen; Grouper; Butterfish; Halibut; Lingcod; Rockfish; Salmon (smoked, Lox); Perch; Boar meat; Rabbit meat; Pheasant; Duck (no skin); Veal shoulder/leg/sirloin; Veal tongue; Cusk; Dolphinfish (Mahi-Mahi); Sturgeon; Sheepshead; Cisco; Seatrout; Turkey breast; Beef; Veal; Snail; Lobster; White fish (smoked); Beef jerky sticks; Pumpkinseed sunfish; Flatfish (flounder & sole); Tilapia; Canned tuna; Turkey dark meat; Pork; Lamb leg; Crayfish; Corned beef; Scallops; Cod; Turbot; Haddock; Northern pike; Orange roughy; Catfish; Bison/buffalo meat; Guinea hen; Eel; Chicken dark meat; Goose;

Eggs, Beans, Nuts and Seeds

Pigeon peas; Split peas; Soy milk; Soybean seeds; Seeds: chia, flaxseed, sunflower, safflower; Soybeans (green); Peanuts; Cottonseed; Almonds; Pistachio nuts; Sesame seeds; Walnuts; Pine nuts; Fava beans; Hazelnuts or Filberts; Egg yolk; Pinto & Navy beans; Lentils; Duck & goose egg; Butternuts; Ginkgo nuts; Beechnuts; Breadnut tree seeds; Black beans; Chickpeas; Black-eyed peas; Green peas; Egg; Cashew nuts; Egg white; various beans; Breadfruit seeds; Watermelon seeds; Hickory nuts; Pecans; Lupin; Pumpkin & squash seeds; Alfalfa sprouts; Sugar or snap peas; Chestnuts; Acorns; Brazil nuts; Cornnuts;

Fruits & Juices

Prunes (dried); Goji berry; Dried banana; Durian; Dried longans; Plantains; Tamarind; Currants (dried); Dried fruits: Litchi, Figs, Peaches; Kiwi fruit; Dried pears; Avocado; Raisins; Blackberries; Passion fruit; Dates; Boysenberries; Elderberries; Guava; Dried fruits; Pineapple juice; Abiyuch; Kumquats; Loganberry; Pomegranate; Raspberries; Rhubarb; Rowal; Olives; Mango; Prune juice; Blueberries and Bilberries; Breadfruit; Cranberries; Currants (raw); Figs; Berries; Grapes; Pears; Pomegranate juice; Banana; Acerola; Apple juice; Apples; Apricots; Cantaloupe; Cherries; Cranberry juice; Grape juice; Honeydew melon; Jujube (fruit); Litchi; Longans; Natal Plum (Carissa); Nectarine; Papaya; Peaches; Persimmons; Pineapple; Pitanga; Plum; Quince; Strawberries; Watermelon;

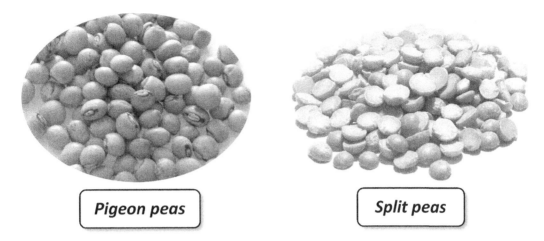

Pigeon peas

Split peas

Vegetables

Shitake mushrooms; Pasilla & Ancho peppers; Sun-dried tomatoes; Balsam pear leafy tips; Grape leaves; Taro leaves; Fungi cloud ears; Winged beans leaves; Chrysanthemum (Garland); Spinach; Turnip greens; Sweet potatoes leaves; Dandelion Greens; Kelp; Collards; Garden cress; Epazote; Savoy cabbage; Endive; Asparagus; Chicory greens; Mustard greens; Amaranth leaves; Romaine lettuce; Chinese broccoli; Beet greens; Arugula; Kale; Pokeberry shoots; Arrowroot; Green onions (scallions); Green & Red cabbage (juice in particular); Okra; Chrysanthemum Leaves; Swiss chard; Jalapeno peppers; Cowpeas leafy tips; Artichoke; Wasabi root; Loose leaf lettuce; Watercress; Bok choy; Leeks; Garlic; Quinoa seed; Potato; Potatoes w/skin; Mustard spinach; Red hot chili peppers; Vine spinach (Basella); Parsnips; Yam; Lambsquarters; Cauliflower; Lotus root; various peppers; Shallots; Sweet potatoes; Broccoli (sprouts in particular); Red bell peppers; Taro; other vegetables;

Breads, Grains, Cereals, Pasta

Wheat bran; Durum wheat; Whole-wheat; Wheat germ cereal; Wheat germ; Amaranth; Rye; Buckwheat; Rice bran; Wheat germ bread; Bran flakes cereal; Whole-wheat cereal; Whole-wheat bread; Corn bran; Triticale; Wheat bran muffins; Whole-wheat spaghetti; Whole-wheat English muffins; Oatmeal (cereal); Shredded wheat cereal; Whole-wheat crackers; Sorghum; Oats; Wheat crackers; Toasted bread; Granola cereal; Corn flakes; Whole-wheat dinner rolls; Oat bran bread; Italian bread; Spelt (cooked); Rice crisps; Pumpernickel bread; Brown rice; Wild rice; Bread sticks; Barley; Bulgur; Saltines crackers; Millet; Chinese chow Mein noodles; Hamburger & hot dog rolls; White bread; Melba toasts crackers; Corn; Oat bran muffins; Waffles; Banana bread; English muffins; Bagels; Cornbread; Corn muffins; Oat bran; French rolls; Pasta; White rice; Matzo crackers; Kaiser dinner rolls; Semolina; Cream of wheat; Milk crackers; Rice cakes (Brown rice based); Tortillas (corn); Spaghetti;

Dairy Products, Fats & Oils

Wheat germ oil; Whey (dried); Canola oil; Yogurt; Cod liver fish oil; various fish oils; Soybean oil; Flaxseed oil;

Desserts, Snacks, Beverages

Air-popped Popcorn; Pretzels; Oil popped popcorn; Honey (Manuka honey in particular); Sesame crunch candies; Ice cream cones; Halvah; Peanut bar candies; Potato chips/fried snacks; Peanut butter; Molasses; Tortilla chips;

Herbs & Spices, Fast Foods, Prepared Foods

Whole-grain cornmeal; Tofu; Cottonseed meal; Tempeh; Teriyaki sauce; Fried tofu; Soy sauce; Miso; Croutons; Thyme (fresh); Natto; Parsley; Hamburger; Basil (fresh); Egg rolls (veg); Coriander/Cilantro; Potato pancakes; Cheeseburger; Peppermint; French fries; Cayenne (red) pepper; Rosemary (fresh); Malt syrup; Taco shells; Spearmint (fresh); Maple syrup; Hush puppies; Sofrito sauce; Cinnamon (helps stomach ulcer in particular); Cole slaw; Dill weed; Sage; Maple sugar;

Alternative Therapies & Miscellaneous

Consult your doctor (check for H. Pylori bacteria); Exercise; Biofeedback; Elimination diet (to determine your food allergies); Socialize, join a club; Antacids;

Key Nutrients & Herbal Medicines

Slippery Elm (for stomach ulcer in particular); DHEA (dehydroepiandosterone); Ginkgo Biloba; Licorice (use in paste form); Omega-3 fatty acids; SAMe (works best with Vitamin B-12 and Folic acid); St. John's wort (a dose of 2-4 grams of the herb for a mild antidepressant action or nervous disturbances); Valerian (don't combine with alcohol);

Do not choose these for Ulcers & Depression

Top 5 items to avoid:

> Alcohol & Smoking; Prescription drugs & Aspirin; Chocolate; Hydrogenated Vegetable Oil; Stress;

Avoid or consume much less of the following (within a food group, most harmful items are listed first):

Meat, Fish & Poultry

Blood sausage; Beef and pork frankfurters; Beef & pork luncheon meats; various sausages;

Instead choose: Chicken wings; Cured beef; Pork headcheese; Bacon; Beef chuck/brisket; Salami; Croaker; Chicken & turkey frankfurter; Lamb tongue; Lamb; Beef tongue; Chorizo; Beef shank; Squab; Cured meats;

Eggs, Beans, Nuts and Seeds

Coconut milk; Coconut;

Instead choose: Lima beans; Egg substitute; Macadamia nuts; Pili nuts;

Fruits & Juices

Grapefruit; Grapefruit juice; Orange juice; Oranges; Pumelo (Shaddock); Tangerines; Lemon; Lime;

Breads, Grains, Cereals, Pasta

There are no items in this food group that would worsen your conditions.

Instead choose: Biscuits; Wheat; Granola bars; Sweet rolls; Blueberry muffins; Japanese noodles; Spinach spaghetti; Couscous; Egg & Rice noodles; Donuts;

Dairy Products, Fats & Oils

Hydrogenated vegetable oil; Chocolate milk; Lard; Animal fat; Margarine; Oils: sesame, Cupu Assu, Shea nut, tea seed, Ucuhuba Butter; Cream; Whipped cream; Butter; Cocoa Butter oil; Poultry fat; Avocado oil; Cream cheese; Margarine-like spreads; various seeds/nuts/vegetable oils; Milk (need to determine if you have allergy to milk); American cheese;

Instead choose: Cottage cheese; Walnut oil; Parmesan cheese; Olive oil; Coconut oil; Mustard oil; Cheeses: Gjetost, Gruyere, Swiss, Camembert, Edam, Limburger, Roquefort, Goat;

Desserts, Snacks, Beverages

80+ proof distilled alcoholic beverages; Whiskey; Coffee liqueur; Crème de menthe; Dark chocolate; Sweet chocolate; Piña colada; Red wine; White wine; Chocolate mousse; Hot chocolate; Chocolate ice cream; Chocolate chip cookies; Chocolate (avoid if it bothers you); Dessert toppings; Beer; Butter cookies; Chocolate cake; Pound cake; After-dinner mints; Coffee; Coconut cream pie; Cheesecake;

Instead <u>*choose*</u>: *Cookies: lady fingers, molasses; Pecan pie; Water; Pumpkin pie; Frostings; Animal crackers; Caramel candies; Peanut brittle candies; Sponge cake; Gingersnaps cookies; Angel food cake; Shortcake; Frozen yogurt; Applesauce; Fruit punch; Ginger ale; Lemonade; Herbal tea; Tonic water;*

Herbs & Spices, Fast Foods, Prepared Foods

Chocolate syrup; Cheese sauce; Nutmeg (avoid if it bothers you); Table sugar (white or powder); Horseradish; Pepper (black or white; avoid if it bothers you);

Instead <u>*choose*</u>: *Oregano; Sorghum syrup; Corn cakes; Tomato paste; Sweet pickle; Chervil; Hummus; Falafel; Breaded shrimp; Cheese fondue; Beef broth; Beef stock; Veg/beef soup; Tarragon (dried); Mustard; Poppy seed; Succotash; Pickle (cucumber); Pizza; Hash brown potatoes; French toast; Cloves; Macaroni; Italian salad dressing; Cardamom; Mints; Sauerkraut; Turmeric; Fish sauce; Hot dog; Onion rings; Chicken Nuggets;*

Alternative Therapies & Miscellaneous

Alcoholic beverages; Smoking, tobacco; Prescription drugs (NSAID and NSAID containing drugs); Aspirin (& other NSAID drugs such as ibuprofen & naproxen); Fasting (for a specific period); Stress; Food allergens (need to determine if food allergies are causing problem);

Key Nutrients & Herbal Medicines

Alcohol; Buckthorn (Herb); Marijuana; Saturated fat;

Diabetes Type 2 & Ulcers

Diabetes is a disorder that refers to our body's inability to use or convert food to the fuel needed by our cells.

Insulin is a hormone that helps the glucose (sugar) get into the body cells. In diabetes, the body is unable to create or properly use insulin. Without insulin, glucose stays in the blood and eventually makes its way to the urine, instead of serving as fuel to our muscles, tissues and brain.

There are different types of diabetes but the most common one is Diabetes Type 2 which represents 90-95% of diabetes cases, and is the focus of this section.

You are at most risk to develop diabetes Type 2 if you are obese. Your risk increases as you get older, if you are a member of a US minority group, are physically inactive, have a family history of the disease, have high blood pressure, have low level of good cholesterol, or have a high level of triglycerides.

Over time, excessive blood sugar level can cause serious health problems, in particular heart related issues. Over 65% of those with diabetes die from heart disease or stroke.

While there is no cure for diabetes type 2, there are numerous tools such as nutrition and exercise to help with the management of this disorder. In addition to managing the blood sugar level, the goal of diabetes management includes control of blood pressure, and cholesterol levels.

Choose these for Diabetes (Type 2) & Ulcers

Top 5 items to choose:

Cabbage/Green leafy vegetables; Whole Grains; Mushrooms; Sun-dried tomatoes; Prunes;

Food items and actions that could improve your health (within a food group, most helpful items are listed first):

Meat, Fish & Poultry

Oysters; Alaskan king crab; Liver; Veal shank; Cured beef; Beef filet mignon; Beef round steak; Turkey & chicken liver; Ground beef; Anchovy; Spiny lobster; Beef rib eye; Beef top sirloin; Sardines; Cuttlefish; Carp; Pout; Smelt; White fish; Chicken breast (no skin); Pork cured/ham; Quail; Pork loin/sirloin; Beef tenderloin/T-bone/portrhse; Marlin; Swordfish; Seabass; Bluefish; Catfish; Cisco (smoked); Cusk; Drum; Flatfish (flounder & sole); Grouper; Halibut; Ling; King mackerel; Milkfish; Monkfish; Mullet; Salmon (smoked, Lox); Pink salmon; Scup; Shad; Shark; Snapper; Spot; Sturgeon; Sucker; Surimi; Tilapia; Tilefish; Trout; various types of tuna; White fish (smoked); Whiting; Wolffish; Yellowtail; Perch; Cisco; Herring; Chicken dark meat; Pollock; Eel; Bison/buffalo meat; Striped bass; Northern pike; Freshwater bass; Rockfish; Pumpkinseed sunfish; Chicken wings; Pork back ribs; Croaker; Veal shoulder/leg/sirloin; Cod; Pheasant; Lingcod; Butterfish; Seatrout; Mackerel; Pompano fish; Sablefish; Sheepshead; Dolphinfish (Mahi-Mahi); Lamb leg; Burbot; Haddock; Orange roughy; Walleye; Goose; Pork shldr; Dungeness crab; Bacon; Turbot; Caviar; Boar meat; Mussels; Snail; Duck (no skin); Octopus; Beef chuck/brisket; Clams; Guinea hen; Veal loin; Fish roe; Venison; Turkey breast; Pork leg/ham; Meatless sausage; Rabbit meat; Turkey dark meat; Whelk; Blue crab; Abalone; Scallops; Beef jerky sticks; Lobster; Beef shank; Beef ribs; Squab (pigeon);

Eggs, Beans, Nuts and Seeds

Pine nuts; Soy milk; Split peas; Soybean seeds; Chia seeds; Flaxseed; Almonds; Fava beans; Sunflower seeds; Soybeans (green); Safflower seeds; Hazelnuts or Filberts; Green peas; Breadnut tree seeds; Peanuts; Cashew nuts; Watermelon seeds; Black walnuts; Beans: black, navy, yellow & white; Chickpeas; Pistachio nuts; Hyacinth beans; Sesame seeds; Pecans; Pumpkin & squash seeds; Black-eyed peas; Pinto beans; Sugar or snap peas; various beans; Cottonseed; Cornnuts; Butternuts; Hickory nuts; Ginkgo nuts; Alfalfa sprouts; Brazil nuts; Walnuts; Acorns; Beechnuts; Lupin; Egg yolk; Breadfruit seeds; Pili nuts; Macadamia nuts; Lentils; Chestnuts; Egg white; Coconut meat (dried); Duck & goose eggs;

Fruits & Juices _(avoid fruit juices with added sugar or from concentrate)_

Prunes (dried); Passion fruit; Dried peaches; Plantains; Avocado; Dried apricots; Elderberries; Guava; Olives; Goji berry; Blackberries; Kumquats; Apricots; Cantaloupe; Mango; Persimmons; Pitanga; Papaya; Raspberries; Abiyuch; Kiwi fruit; Rowal; Acerola; Durian; Dried banana; Gooseberries; Watermelon; Berries; Cranberries; Dried figs; Jujube (fruit); Rhubarb; Dried fruits; Apples; Currants (raw); Pears; Banana; Strawberries; Peaches; Nectarine; Plum; Natal Plum (Carissa); Currants (dried); Pomegranate; Raisins; Dates; Breadfruit; Tamarind; Blueberries and Bilberries; Pineapple; Apple juice; Figs; Honeydew melon; Cherries; Pomegranate juice; Quince; Grape juice; Litchi; Grapes; Cranberry juice; Prune juice; Longans; Pineapple juice; Grapefruit; Lemon; Lime;

Vegetables

Grape leaves; Shitake mushrooms; Sun-dried tomatoes; Pigeon peas; Sweet potatoes leaves; Green & Red cabbages (juice in particular); Dandelion Greens; Beet greens; Chicory greens; Collards; Mustard greens; Taro leaves; Turnip greens; Chinese broccoli; Savoy cabbage; Chrysanthemum (Garland); Endive; Fungi cloud ears; Green onions (scallions); Ancho & Pasilla peppers; Spinach; Swiss chard; Amaranth leaves; Arugula; Balsam pear leafy tips; Garden cress; Kale; Romaine & loose leaf lettuce; Pokeberry shoots; Watercress; Asparagus; Bok choy; Leeks; Okra; Wasabi root; Parsnips; Jalapeno peppers; Carrots; Green beans; Kelp; Cauliflower; Chrysanthemum Leaves; Mustard spinach; Sweet potatoes; Winged beans leaves; Red & green bell peppers; Kohlrabi; Borage; Celtuce; Hot chili peppers; Pimento peppers; Potato; Pumpkin; Pumpkin flowers; Purslane; Winter squash; Tahitian taro; Tomatoes; Vine spinach (Basella); Banana peppers; Epazote; Quinoa seed; Cowpeas leafy tips; Lambsquarters; Portabella mushrooms; Broccoli (sprouts in particular); Brussels sprouts; Yam; other vegetables;

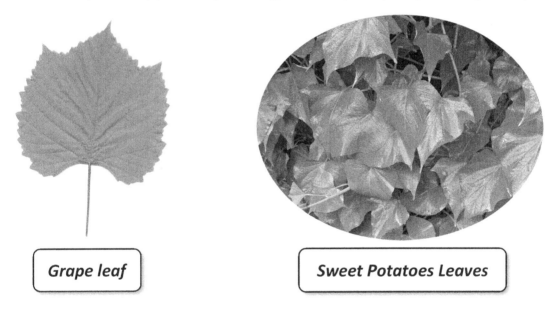

Grape leaf   **Sweet Potatoes Leaves**

Breads, Grains, Cereals, Pasta

Rye; Corn bran; Durum wheat; Whole-wheat; Buckwheat; Amaranth; Whole-wheat cereal; Wheat germ cereal; Whole-wheat English muffins; Triticale; Whole-wheat spaghetti; Wheat germ; Sorghum; Spelt (cooked); Wheat bran muffins; Rice bran; Wild rice; Whole-wheat crackers; Oatmeal (cereal); Wheat germ bread; Whole-wheat dinner rolls; Bulgur; Oats; Millet; Shredded wheat; Granola cereal; Pumpernickel bread; Chinese chow Mein noodles; Rice cakes (Brown rice based); Toasted bread; Corn; Whole-wheat bread (whole-grains only); Banana bread; Corn flakes; Rice crisps cereal; Bread sticks; Barley; Italian bread; Wheat crackers; Oat bran muffins; Brown rice; Tortillas (corn); Cream of wheat; Oat bran bread; English muffins; Wheat; Biscuits; Bagels; Semolina; Oat bran; Waffles; Granola bars; White rice; Spaghetti; Pasta; Wheat bran; Corn muffins; Melba toasts crackers;

Dairy Products, Fats & Oils

Wheat germ oil; Canola oil; Margarine; Olive oil; Margarine-like spreads; Oils: hazelnut, safflower, almonds, grape seeds, soybean, apricot kernel; Cod liver fish oil; various seeds/nuts/vegetable oils; Cottage cheese; Yogurt; Cheese: parmesan, Gruyere; Salmon fish oil; Edam & Swiss cheese; Cheese spread; Fontina cheese; Sesame oil;

Desserts, Snacks, Beverages

Air Popped Popcorn; Oil popped Popcorn; Sesame crunch candies; Tortilla chips; Potato chips/fried snacks; Peanut butter; Taro chips; Potato sticks; Peanut bar candies; Pretzels; Water; Pumpkin pie;

Herbs & Spices, Fast Foods, Prepared Foods

Whole-grain Cornmeal; Tofu; Coriander/Cilantro; Parsley; Basil (fresh); Cottonseed meal; Thyme (fresh); Cayenne (red) pepper; Natto; Rosemary (fresh); Peppermint; Fried tofu; Spearmint (fresh); Tomato paste; Poppy seed; French fries; Egg rolls (veg); Tempeh; Soups: minestrone, vegetable, veg/beef; Dill weed; Taco shells; Mayonnaise; Hash brown potatoes; Mace; Corn salad; Miso; Croutons; Falafel; Cinnamon (for stomach ulcer in particular); Mustard seed (avoid only if it bothers you); Onion rings; Cloves; Oregano; Foie gras or liver pate; Potato pancakes; Hummus; Cole slaw; French salad dressing; Sage; Maple sugar; Succotash; Tarragon (dried); Teriyaki sauce; Cheese fondue; Blue/Roquefort salad dressing; Chervil; Mustard; Cardamom; Sweet pickle; Chives; Mints; Pickle relish;

Alternative Therapies & Miscellaneous

Consult your doctor (check for H. Pylori bacteria; for diabetes maintain annual physical exam, get vaccinated, monitor eyes, foot, blood pressure ...); Eat smaller, more frequent meals; Exercise; Biofeedback; Elimination diet (to determine possible food allergies); Glucomannan; Antacids; Exposure to sun;

Key Nutrients & Herbal Medicines

Fiber (soluble fiber in particular); Slippery Elm (for stomach ulcer in particular); Zinc; Brewer's Yeast; Chromium; Monounsaturated fat; Polyunsaturated fat; Siberian Ginseng; Gymnema; Licorice (in paste form); Vitamin A; Beta Carotene; Vitamin E; Fenugreek seeds;

Do not choose these for Ulcers & Diabetes (Type 2)

Top 5 items to avoid:

Fasting; Chocolate; Sugar & Sweets; Animal Fat; Alcohol & Smoking;

Avoid or consume much less of the following (within a food group, most harmful items are listed first):

Meat, Fish & Poultry

Pepperoni; Pastrami; Chicken skin; Turkey skins; Blood sausage; Beerwurst beer salami; Frankfurters; Luncheon meats; Bologna; Sausages; Cured beef; Chorizo; Salami; Lamb brain; Veal thymus; Beef tongue;

Instead choose: Lamb shoulder; Ground lamb; Lamb loin; Veal tongue; Corned beef; Shrimp; Crayfish;

Eggs, Beans, Nuts and Seeds

Coconut milk; Coconut; Egg substitute;

Fruits & Juices

Avoid sugared juices or made from concentrate;

Breads, Grains, Cereals, Pasta

Danish pastry; Croissant; White bread; Donuts; Sweet rolls; Milk crackers; Bran flakes cereal;

Instead choose: Hamburger & hot dog rolls; Saltines; Spinach spaghetti; Cornbread; Matzo crackers; Japanese noodles; Couscous; various noodles; French rolls; Blueberry muffins; Kaiser dinner rolls;

Dairy Products, Fats & Oils

Animal fat; Hydrogenated vegetable oil; Lard; Chocolate milk; Whipped cream; Cream; Poultry fat; Ucuhuba Butter oil; Sour cream; Coconut oil; Whey (dried); Non-dairy creamers; Skim milk; American cheese; Milk (determine if you have allergy to milk); Fat-free or low fat products;

Instead choose: Cheese: goat, cheddar, Colby, camembert, pimento, Gjetost, gouda; Herring fish oil; Vegetable shortening; Blue cheese; Port de Salut cheese; Ricotta cheese; Limburger cheese; Sardine fish oil; Babassu oil; Brie cheese; Mozzarella cheese; Menhaden fish oil; Cream cheese; Romano cheese;

Desserts, Snacks, Beverages

Sweet chocolate; Coffee liqueur; Chocolate ice cream; Dark chocolate; Chocolate mousse; Chocolate chip cookies; Crème de menthe; Pound cake; Butter cookies; Vanilla ice cream; Dessert toppings; various cakes; various cookies; Frozen yogurt; After-dinner mints; Cheesecake; Pudding; Éclairs; Piña colada; various pies; Cream puffs; Fruit leather/rolls; Soft (carbonated) drinks; various candies; Hot chocolate; 80+ proof distilled alcoholic beverages; Whiskey; Chewing gum; Jams & Preserves; Jellies; Sherbet; Fruit punch; Lemonade; Ice cream cones; Molasses; Coffee; Puff pastry; Frostings; Pancakes; Red & white wine; Eggnog; Plain tea (avoid if bothers you); Coffeecake; Milk shakes; Malted drinks (nonalcoholic); Honey (if you must have it choose Manuka honey); Beer;

Instead _choose_: Halvah; Herbal tea;

Herbs & Spices, Fast Foods, Prepared Foods

Chocolate syrup; Table sugar (white or powder); Barbecue sauce; various syrups; Cheese sauce; Hot dog; Hoisin sauce; Nutmeg (avoid if it bothers you); Ketchup; Nachos; various sauces; Chicken Nuggets; Tabasco sauce; Brown sugar; Pizza; Horseradish; Cheeseburger; Tapioca;

Instead _choose_: Sauerkraut; Cocoa; Turmeric; Fennel seeds; Pickle (cucumber); Soy sauce; Corn cakes; Beef broth; Beef stock; Clam chowder; Fish stock; Ginger; Saffron; Hush puppies; Hamburger; Chicken stock; Chicken broth; Chicken noodle soup; Italian salad dressing; Capers; Gravies; Marjoram; Pepper (Black or white; avoid if bothers you); Table salt; Vinegar; Potato salad;

Alternative Therapies & Miscellaneous

Fasting (for a specific period); Alcoholic beverages; Smoking, tobacco; Stress; Prescription drugs (NSAID containing drugs); Aspirin (& other NSAID drugs); Excess body weight; Fried or battered foods; Corn sweetener; Processed or Refined foods; Baking using butter; Sweeteners; Abrupt changes in diet/exercise; Food allergens (need to determine your food allergies); Aspartame (Equal); Saccharine (NutraSweet);

Key Nutrients & Herbal Medicines

Alcohol; Saturated fat; Refined sugar; Caffeine; Buckthorn (Herb); Cholesterol; Total sugar; Trans fatty acids; Guarana; Kola (cola); Mate;

Excess Body Weight or Obesity & Ulcers

Obesity is defined as having too much body fat. It normally occurs when you continue to eat more calories than your body burns through exercise and normal daily activities. The unused calories are then stored as fat in your body leading to obesity.

Obesity is a risk factor for many diseases and illnesses including certain types of cancer. However, even a modest reduction in body fat (5 to 10% weight loss) can reduce your risk or delay illnesses caused by obesity.

The common way to measure obesity is body mass index (BMI). BMI is calculated by multiplying your weight in pounds by 703, divided by the square of your height in inches. For example a 6 feet tall man who weighs 190 pounds, has a BMI of 25.8. In the metric system, BMI is your weight in kilograms divided by the square of your height in meters.

Your BMI is considered normal if it is between 18.5 and 24.9. You are obese if your BMI is 30 or higher. You have excess body weight if your BMI is between 24.9 and 30.

Risk factors that can lead to obesity include: lack of physical exercise, overeating (e.g., oversized portions, recovery from quitting smoking), poor diet (e.g., eating high-fat foods), genetic or family history, pregnancy (inability to lose weight after giving birth), hormone problems, certain medications and illnesses, emotional issues (boredom, anger or stress), growing older, and lack of sleep.

Choose these for Ulcers & Excess Body Weight

Top 5 items to choose:

**Green leafy vegetables; Mushrooms; Peas;
Whole Grains; Passion fruit & Berries;**

Food items and actions that could improve your health (within a food group, most helpful items are listed first):

Meat, Fish & Poultry

(5.5 oz. of meat/fowl/fish or beans per day); Surimi; Seabass; Cisco; Cod; Cusk; Grouper; Ling; Monkfish; Northern pike; Shark; Snapper; Sucker; Tilapia; Yellowfin tuna; Wolffish; Pout; Pumpkinseed sunfish; Orange roughy; Freshwater bass; Burbot; Catfish; Halibut; Lingcod; King mackerel; Rockfish; Scup; Seatrout; Sheepshead; Sturgeon; Tilefish; Turbot; Whiting; Perch; Smelt; Flatfish (flounder & sole); Pink salmon; Blue fin tuna; Canned tuna; Striped bass; Dolphinfish (Mahi-Mahi); Walleye pike; Pollock;

Eggs, Beans, Nuts and Seeds

(5.5 oz. of meat/fowl/fish or beans per day); Split peas; Beans: fava, black, navy, yellow & white; Lentils; Chickpeas; Alfalfa sprouts; Mung & Pinto beans; Green peas; various beans; Black-eyed peas; Soybeans (green); Sugar or snap peas; Lupin; Soybean seeds; Soy milk; Chia seeds; Breadnut tree seeds;

Fruits & Juices

(2 cups of fruits & juices per day; favor fruits over juices; drink fruit juice before meals); Passion fruit; Blackberries; Elderberries; Raspberries; Kiwi fruit; Abiyuch; Boysenberries; Guava; Kumquats; Loganberry; Prunes (dried); Rowal; Cranberries; Durian; Gooseberries; Rhubarb; Dried figs; Currants (raw); Pears; Pomegranate; Dried fruits; Avocado; Breadfruit; Plantains; Acerola; various berries; Jujube (fruit); Natal Plum (Carissa); Persimmons; Pitanga; Strawberries; Blueberries; Figs; Apple juice; Apricots; Cantaloupe; Honeydew melon; Nectarine; Papaya; Peaches; Pineapple; Plum; Watermelon; Olives; Pomegranate juice; Banana; Apples; Cherries; Cranberry juice; Grape juice; Mango; Quince; Grapes; Tamarind; Litchi; Prune juice; Goji berry; Currants (dried); Dates; Raisins; Longans; Pineapple juice; Lemon; Lime;

Vegetables

(2.5 cups per day); Grape leaves; Fungi cloud ears; Pigeon peas; Ancho peppers; Shitake mushrooms; Pasilla peppers; Sweet potatoes leaves; Wasabi root; Green cabbage (juice in particular); Dandelion Greens; Beet greens; Chicory greens; Collards; Mustard greens; Taro leaves; Turnip greens; Chinese broccoli; Savoy cabbage; Chrysanthemum (Garland); Endive; Green onions (scallions); Red cabbage (juice in particular); Sun-dried tomatoes; Artichoke; Kelp; Jalapeno peppers; Spinach; Swiss chard; Amaranth leaves; Arugula; Balsam pear leafy tips; Garden cress; Kale; Romaine & loose leaf lettuce; Okra; Pokeberry shoots; Watercress; Quinoa seed; Asparagus; Parsnips; Yam; Carrots; Epazote; Green beans; Bok choy; Leeks; Taro; Balsam pear; Chrysanthemum Leaves; Eggplant; Fennel; Kohlrabi; Lotus root; Mustard spinach; various peppers; Potato; Sweet potatoes; Celery; Head lettuce; Shallots; Cauliflower; Cucumbers with peel; Winged beans leaves; Red bell peppers; Arrowhead; Arrowroot; Green bell peppers; Borage; Celtuce; Cowpeas leafy tips; Fiddlehead ferns; various mushrooms; other vegetables;

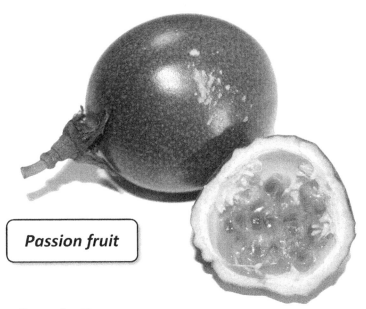

Passion fruit

Breads, Grains, Cereals, Pasta

(6 oz. of grains per day with over 3 oz. from whole grains); Corn bran; Rye; Durum wheat; Buckwheat; Whole-wheat cereal; Amaranth; Spelt (cooked); Barley; Bulgur; Sorghum; Wild rice; Whole-wheat spaghetti; Millet; Brown rice; Wheat germ cereal; Triticale; Oatmeal (cereal); Whole-wheat bread; Whole-wheat English muffins; Oats; Rice bran; Corn; Whole-wheat; Oat bran; Shredded wheat cereal; Wheat bran; English muffins; White rice; Bran flakes cereal;

Dairy Products, Fats & Oils

(3 cups of low fat products per day); Fat-free/Low fat dairy products; Yogurt;

Desserts, Snacks, Beverages

Air-popped popcorn; Water;

Herbs & Spices, Fast Foods, Prepared Foods

Whole-grain Cornmeal; Thyme (fresh); Rosemary (fresh); Tofu; Peppermint; Coriander/Cilantro; Parsley; Cayenne (red) pepper; Cinnamon (stomach ulcer in particular); Spearmint (fresh); Basil (fresh); Natto; Cole slaw; Tempeh;

Alternative Therapies & Miscellaneous

Consult your doctor (check for H. Pylori); Exercise (including sit-ups and lower back exercises); Antacids; Choose smaller food portions & meals; Elimination diet (need to determine which foods cause problems for your ulcer); Hang mirrors where you eat; Walk, wheel, or jog (suck stomach in while running);

Key Nutrients & Herbal Medicines

Fiber; Slippery Elm (for stomach ulcer in particular); Licorice (use in paste form; for Ulcers);

Do not choose these for Ulcers & Excess Body Weight

Top 5 items to avoid:

Chocolate; 2+ alcoholic drinks/day; Cheese;
Cream & Butter; Luncheon (processed) Meats;

Avoid or consume much less of the following (within a food group, most harmful items are listed first):

Meat, Fish & Poultry

Blood sausage; Pepperoni; Frankfurters; Luncheon meats; Chorizo; various sausage; Pastrami; various salami; Pork skins; Poultry skins; Pork liver cheese; Bacon; Pork breakfast strips; Pork ribs; Lamb ribs; Bologna; Pork spare ribs; Caviar; Cured beef; Beef ribs; Beef tongue; Lamb loin; Lamb tongue; Lamb; Pork; Beef; Beef jerky sticks; Squab (pigeon); Cured meats; Pancreas (lamb, beef, veal); Bison/buffalo meat; Veal tongue; Eel; Goose; Organ meats; Chicken & turkey liver; Calamari; Chicken wings; Shrimp; Corned beef; Veal loin; Chicken dark meat; Liver; Whelk; Rabbit meat; Mackerel; Sablefish; Venison; Beef filet mignon; Veal shoulder/leg/sirloin; Clams; Boar meat; Fish roe; Pompano fish; Abalone;

Instead **choose**: Oysters; Bluefish; Drum; Haddock; Mullet; Spot; Carp; White fish; Marlin; Swordfish; Butterfish; Milkfish; Trout; Yellowtail; Quail breast; Spiny lobster; White fish (smoked); Chicken breast (no skin); Cisco (smoked); Salmon (smoked, Lox); Pheasant breast; Snail; Turkey breast; Dungeness crab; Alaskan king crab; Shad; Cuttlefish; Guinea hen; Herring; Turkey dark meat; Sardines;

Eggs, Beans, Nuts and Seeds

Coconut milk; Pili nuts; Coconut; Egg yolk; Macadamia nuts; Brazil nuts; Walnuts; Coconut meat (dried); Cottonseed; Hickory nuts; Pumpkin & squash seeds; Beechnuts; Cashew nuts; Watermelon seeds; Egg substitute; Acorns; Butternuts; Pecans; Peanuts; Pistachio nuts; Cornnuts; Hazelnuts or Filberts; Egg (no more than four per week); Egg white; Pine nuts; Sunflower seeds;

Instead **choose**: Flaxseed; Breadfruit seeds; Almonds;

Fruits & Juices

Avoid sugared juices and those made from concentrate;

Breads, Grains, Cereals, Pasta

Croissant; Milk crackers; Sweet rolls; Donuts; Granola bars; Danish pastry; Rice crisps cereal; Saltines crackers; Blueberry muffins; Granola cereal; Biscuits; Wheat crackers; Kaiser dinner rolls; Corn flakes; French rolls; Matzo crackers; Melba toasts crackers; Bread sticks; Waffles; White bread; Hamburger & hot dog rolls; Banana bread; Chinese chow Mein noodles; Cornbread; Wheat;

Instead **choose**: Tortillas (corn); Whole-wheat crackers; Whole-wheat dinner rolls; Wheat germ bread; Pumpernickel bread; Pasta; Spaghetti; Bagels; Couscous; various noodles; Spinach spaghetti; Rice cakes (Brown rice based); Oat bran bread; Wheat germ;

Dairy Products, Fats & Oils

Cream cheese; Goat cheese; Cream; Whipped cream; Cheese: Gjetost, Limburger, Roquefort; Butter; Cheese spread; various cheese; Animal fat; Lard; Sesame oil; Poultry fat; Whey (dried); Oils: coconut, Cupu Assu, Shea nut, tea seed, Ucuhuba Butter, Cocoa Butter, tomato seeds; Sour cream; Chocolate milk; Hydrogenated vegetable oil; various seeds/nuts/vegetable oils; Vegetable shortening; Sardine fish oil; Margarine-like spreads; Menhaden fish oil; Margarine; Olive oil; various fish oil; Non-dairy creamers; Canola oil; Wheat germ oil; Salmon fish oil; Milk;

Instead <u>**choose**</u>**: Low fat & low salt cottage cheese;**

Desserts, Snacks, Beverages

Sweet chocolate; Dark chocolate; Chocolate ice cream; Chocolate mousse; Coffee liqueur; Chocolate chip cookies; Pound cake; various cookies; Vanilla ice cream; Dessert toppings; various cakes; Frozen yogurt; After-dinner mints; Cheesecake; Puff pastry; Crème de menthe; Éclairs; Pie crust; various pies; Cream puffs; Fruit leather/rolls; Coffeecake; Carob candies; Potato sticks; Chewing gum; Ice cream cones; Jams & Preserves; Jellies; Taro chips; Sherbet; various candies; Pancakes; Fruit punch; Lemonade; Molasses; Frostings; Hot chocolate; Peanut butter; Pudding; 80+ proof distilled alcoholic beverages; Whiskey; Tortilla chips; Piña colada; Soft (carbonated) drinks; Coffee; Pretzels; Potato chips/fried snacks; Milk shakes; Red & white wine; Eggnog; Plain tea (avoid if it bothers you); Honey (choose Manuka honey); Malted drinks (nonalcoholic); Beer;

Instead <u>**choose**</u>**: Herbal tea; Applesauce; Green tea;**

Herbs & Spices, Fast Foods, Prepared Foods

Chocolate syrup; Cheese sauce; Table sugar (white or powder); Nachos; Foie gras or liver pate; Hot dog; Pizza; Barbecue sauce; Chicken Nuggets; Hoisin sauce; Sofrito sauce; Ketchup; Blue/Roquefort salad dressing; Fish sauce; Oyster sauce; various syrups; Italian salad dressing; French salad dressing; Mayonnaise; Tapioca; Soy sauce; Tabasco sauce; Cheese fondue; Onion rings; Cheeseburger; French toast; Cocoa; Breaded shrimp; Falafel; Nutmeg (avoid if bothers you); Brown sugar; Hash brown potatoes; Corn cakes; Potato pancakes; Teriyaki sauce; Macaroni; Hamburger; Taco shells; Horseradish; Capers; Table salt; Hush puppies; Potato salad; Maple sugar; Mustard seed (avoid if it bothers you);

Instead <u>**choose**</u>**: Oregano; Sage; Cloves; Fennel seeds; Mace; Succotash; Turmeric; Poppy seed; Egg rolls (veg); Sauerkraut; Cottonseed meal; Chervil; Mints; Cardamom; Dill weed; Ginger; Marjoram; Saffron; Tarragon; Vinegar; Pickles;**

Alternative Therapies & Miscellaneous

2+ alcoholic drinks/day; Stress; Aspirin (& other NSAID drugs); Fried or battered foods (if you fry, use polyunsaturated oils); Prescription drugs (avoid NSAID containing drugs); Corn sweetener; Processed or Refined foods; Fasting (for a specific period); Food allergens (determine if food allergy cause problems for your Ulcers); Smoking, tobacco; Baking using butter; Sweeteners;

Key Nutrients & Herbal Medicines

Saturated fat; Refined sugar; Alcohol; Buckthorn (Herb); Caffeine;

Daily calorie intake should be limited to 10 for each pound of your desired weight, e.g., for a desired weight of 160 lbs., consume 1,600 calories per day.

High Blood Pressure & Ulcers

High blood pressure (HBP), also known as Hypertension, is a serious condition and can lead to other health issues such as heart attack, stroke and kidney failure.

Your blood pressure is an indication of how hard your heart has to work to pump blood through your arteries and how much resistance to blood flow exists in your arteries. It is highest when your heart beats, pumping the blood (systolic pressure). And it is the lowest between beats (diastolic pressure).

The blood pressure is often shown in form of a ratio, Systolic/Diastolic pressure, and measured in millimeters of mercury. Your blood pressure is considered normal if the Systolic number is less than 120 and Diastolic number is lower than 80. For example, if your blood pressure numbers are 115/79, you are fine. But if your top number is 140 or higher, or your bottom number is 90 or higher then you have HBP. If your numbers are in between normal and high, then you are likely to end up with HBP unless you take some action to prevent it.

There is no clear cause for HBP among adults. But there are some medical conditions (e.g., kidney problems, sleep apnea), certain medications (e.g., birth control pills) and use of some illegal drugs (e.g., cocaine) that can cause the blood pressure to rise.

You are more likely to develop HBP if you are: an over 55 man, an over 45 woman, black, overweight, physically inactive, under a lot of stress, smoke, drink too much alcohol, eat too much salt/sodium, do not eat enough potassium or Vitamin D, or have a family history of HBP.

Choose these for High Blood Pressure & Ulcers

Top 5 items to choose:

Green leafy vegetables; Whole Grains; Sun-dried tomatoes; Dried fruits; Soy milk;

Food items and actions that could improve your health (within a food group, most helpful items are listed first):

Meat, Fish & Poultry

Snail; Fish roe; White fish; Pink salmon; Whelk; Marlin; Swordfish; Carp; Trout; Snapper; Sardines; Blue fin tuna; Ling; Sturgeon; Perch; Seabass; Catfish; Spiny lobster; Spot; Pout; Monkfish; Tilefish; Smelt; Pollock; Herring; Octopus; Freshwater bass; Halibut; Walleye; Mackerel; Bluefish; King mackerel; Striped bass; Whiting; Oysters; Yellowfin tuna; Yellowtail; Cisco (smoked); Drum; Sucker; Wolffish; Pumpkinseed sunfish; Sheepshead; Mussels; Lingcod; Scup; Milkfish; Burbot; Cusk; Shad; Shark; Dungeness crab; Dolphinfish (Mahi-Mahi); Mullet; Eel; Northern pike; Cuttlefish; Tilapia; Crayfish; Pompano fish; Blue crab; Grouper; Rockfish; Surimi; Veal shank; Cisco; Liver; Calamari; Caviar; Turbot; Alaskan king crab; Butterfish; Seatrout;

Eggs, Beans, Nuts and Seeds

Soy milk; Split peas; Pine nuts; Soybean seeds; Chia seeds; Flaxseed; Almonds; Sunflower seeds; Safflower seeds; Soybeans (green); Hazelnuts or Filberts; Breadnut tree seeds; Fava beans; Cottonseed; Navy beans; Pistachio nuts; Watermelon seeds; various beans; Chickpeas; Lentils; Black walnuts; Breadfruit seeds; Cashew nuts; Pumpkin & squash seeds; Green peas; Butternuts; Ginkgo nuts; Peanuts; Alfalfa sprouts; Brazil nuts; Black-eyed peas; Walnuts; Chestnuts; Sugar or snap peas; Lupin; Pili nuts; Pecans; Sesame seeds; Hickory nuts; Beechnuts; Acorns; Cornnuts;

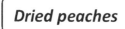
Dried peaches
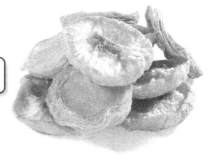

Fruits & Juices

Dried fruits: Prunes, figs, peaches, banana, apricots; Raisins; Tamarind; Currants (dried); Dried litchi; Dried pears; Passion fruit; Dates; Goji berry; dried fruits; Kiwi fruit; Plantains; Abiyuch; Blackberries; Elderberries; Guava; Avocado; Prune juice; Grape juice; Boysenberries; Kumquats; Loganberry; Raspberries; Rowal; Breadfruit; Currants (raw); Durian; Pineapple juice; Cranberry juice; Pears; Pomegranate; Apricots; Cantaloupe; Jujube (fruit); Longans; Natal Plum (Carissa); Persimmons; Figs; Gooseberries; Banana; Apple juice; Grapes; Blueberries; Pomegranate juice; Apples; Peaches; Acerola; Cherries; various berries; Honeydew melon; Litchi; Mango; Nectarine; Papaya; Pineapple; Pitanga; Plum; Quince; Strawberries; Watermelon; Rhubarb; Cranberries; Olives;

Vegetables

Grape leaves; Shitake mushrooms; Sun-dried tomatoes; Pigeon peas; Fungi cloud ears; Ancho & pasilla peppers; Sweet potatoes leaves; Taro leaves; Amaranth leaves; Dandelion Greens; Balsam pear leafy tips; Chrysanthemum (Garland); Wasabi root; Kelp; Garden cress; Kale; Chicory greens; Collards; Mustard greens; Turnip greens; Arugula; Chinese broccoli; Epazote; Artichoke; Beet greens; Watercress; Endive; Green onions (scallions); Okra; Arrowhead; Green cabbage (juice in particular); Spinach; Tahitian taro; Vine spinach (Basella); Red cabbage (juice in particular); Bok choy; Savoy cabbage; Chrysanthemum Leaves; Mustard spinach; Garlic; Taro; Parsnips; Romaine or loose leaf lettuce; Nopal; Pokeberry shoots; Potatoes w/skin; Yam; Asparagus; Carrots; Winged beans leaves; Quinoa seed; Swiss chard; Lotus root; Cauliflower; Balsam pear; Borage; Cowpeas leafy tips; Kohlrabi; Leeks; Purslane; Shallots; Jalapeno peppers; Onions (2-5 oz. of fresh onion daily, or 1 tsp. onion juice 3-4 times a day); Green beans; other vegetables;

Breads, Grains, Cereals, Pasta

Rye; Durum wheat; Whole-wheat; Buckwheat; Corn bran; Amaranth; Wheat bran; Wheat germ cereal; Whole-wheat bread; Wheat germ; Whole-wheat English muffins; Triticale; Whole-wheat cereal; Whole-wheat spaghetti; Sorghum; Rice bran; Oats; Oatmeal (cereal); Wheat bran muffins; Spelt (cooked); Wheat germ bread; Bran flakes cereal; Millet; Brown rice; Barley; Bulgur; Wild rice; Corn; Whole-wheat dinner rolls; Whole-wheat crackers; Oat bran muffins; Shredded wheat; Granola cereal; Oat bran; Rice cakes (Brown rice based); Tortillas (corn); Pumpernickel bread; Toasted bread; Oat bran bread;

Dairy Products, Fats & Oils

What germ oil; Whey (dried); Yogurt; Fat-Free or Low Fat Products;

Desserts, Snacks, Beverages

Air-popped Popcorn; Sesame crunch candies; Molasses; Water; Oil popped popcorn; Honey (Manuka honey for stomach ulcer in particular); Peanut butter;

Herbs & Spices, Fast Foods, Prepared Foods

Whole-grain Cornmeal; Tofu; Cottonseed meal; Thyme (fresh); Natto; Peppermint; Fried tofu; Rosemary (fresh); Parsley; Tempeh; Basil (fresh); Coriander/Cilantro; Spearmint (fresh); Cheese fondue; Cayenne (red) pepper; Cinnamon (for stomach ulcer in particular); Dill weed; Sorghum syrup; Oregano; Tomato paste; Sage; Maple sugar; Miso; Succotash; French fries; Poppy seed; Fennel seeds; Cole slaw; Tarragon (dried); Chervil;

Alternative Therapies & Miscellaneous

Consult your doctor (check for H. Pylori); Follow DASH diet; Antacids; Biofeedback; Elimination diet (to determine which foods cause problems for you); Exercise; Fresh (uncooked) fruits/veg's; Meditation; Ornish Plan & Diet; Pray, practice your religion; Sleep 6-8 hours regularly; Tai Chi; Yoga (certain postures must be avoided); Salt-free or low-salt foods; Organically grown foods;

Key Nutrients & Herbal Meds

Hawthorn (for BHP, in berries form or tea from dried leaves and flowers; do not take with other heart medications); Slippery Elm (for stomach ulcer in particular); Calcium; Celery seed; Fiber; Siberian Ginseng; Magnesium; Potassium; Yucca;

Do not choose these for High Blood Pressure & Ulcers

Top 5 items to avoid:

> Chocolate & Sweets; 2+ alcoholic drinks/day;
> Processed Meats; Caffeine & Smoking; Stress;

Avoid or consume much less of the following (within a food group, most harmful items are listed first):

Meat, Fish & Poultry

Blood sausage; Pepperoni; Beef & pork frankfurters; Beef & pork luncheon meats; Chorizo; Liver sausage; various sausage; various salami; Pork skins; Pork liver cheese; Pork breakfast strips; Bacon; Turkey pastrami; Chicken & turkey frankfurter; Cured beef; Poultry skins; Cured meats; Bologna; various pastrami; Beef jerky sticks; Pork ribs; Pork headcheese; Pork cured/ham; Squab (pigeon); Beef tongue; Lamb ribs; Corned beef; Beef ribs; Lamb tongue; Salmon (smoked, Lox); Beef chuck/brisket; Pork spare ribs; Beef shank; Chicken wings; Lamb loin; Pork back ribs;

Instead _choose_: Anchovy; Flatfish (flounder & sole); Lamb liver; Chicken breast (no skin); Beef filet mignon; Abalone; Scallops; Beef round steak; Cod; Orange roughy; Veal shoulder/leg/sirloin; Haddock; Chicken liver; Rabbit meat; Venison; Canned tuna; Pork loin/sirloin; Turkey dark meat; Ground beef; Boar meat; White fish (smoked); Lobster; Turkey breast; Veal loin; Lamb leg; Quail breast; Duck (no skin); Beef rib eye; Beef top sirloin; Pheasant; Shrimp; Clams; Sablefish; Guinea hen; Croaker;

Eggs, Beans, Nuts and Seeds

Coconut milk;

Instead _choose_: Coconut meat (dried); Macadamia nuts; Egg white; Egg;

Fruits & Juices

Avoid sugared juices or made from concentrate.

Vegetables

Avoid salted canned vegetables.

Breads, Grains, Cereals, Pasta

Croissant; Saltines crackers; Danish pastry; Milk crackers; Sweet rolls; Rice crisps cereal; Donuts; Kaiser dinner rolls; French rolls; Wheat crackers; Biscuits; White bread; Hamburger & hot dog rolls; Waffles; Corn flakes;

Instead _choose_: Semolina; Wheat; Spinach spaghetti; Corn muffins; Cornbread; White rice; Italian bread; Egg noodles; Couscous; various noodles; Pasta; Spaghetti; English muffins; Banana bread;

Dairy Products, Fats & Oils

Chocolate milk; Butter; Brie cheese; Hydrogenated vegetable oil; Roquefort cheese; Goat cheese; Animal fat; Sesame oil; Lard; Pimento cheese; Feta cheese; Oils: Cupu Assu, Shea nut, tea seed, Ucuhuba Butter; Cheese: camembert, cream, limburger; Whipped cream; Cocoa Butter oil; Margarine-like spreads; various cheese; Poultry fats; Margarine; various seeds/nuts/vegetable oils; Cream; Sour cream; Vegetable shortening; Milk (determine if allergic to milk); Olive oil; Ricotta cheese; Soybean oil; Skim milk; Gruyere cheese; Non-dairy creamers;

Instead choose: Cod liver fish oil; Herring fish oil; various fish oil; Flaxseed oil; Cottage cheese; Canola oil; Swiss cheese; Milk shakes; Gjetost cheese;

Desserts, Snacks, Beverages

Sweet chocolate; Chocolate ice cream; Coffee liqueur; Chocolate chip cookie; Pound cake; various cookies; Hot chocolate; Chocolate mousse; Puff pastry; Coffee; Pie crust; Chocolate cake; Dessert toppings; Cheesecake; Éclairs; various cakes; Cream puffs; Vanilla ice cream; Coffeecake; Pretzels; various pies; After-dinner mints; 80+ proof distilled alcoholic beverages; Fruit leather/rolls; Dark chocolate; Pudding; Crème de menthe; Plain tea (avoid if it bothers you); Potato sticks; Piña colada; Soft (carbonated) drinks; Peanut brittle; Ice cream cones; Pancakes; Frostings; Pumpkin pie; Frozen yogurt; Fruit punch; Lemonade; Chewing gum; Jams & Preserves; Sherbet; Green tea;

Instead choose: Potato chips/fried snacks; Tonic water; Tortilla chips; Halvah; Sports drinks; Applesauce; Ginger ale; Herbal tea; Eggnog; Malted drinks (nonalcoholic);

Herbs & Spices, Fast Foods, Prepared Foods

Foie gras or liver pate; Oyster sauce; Chocolate syrup; Cheese sauce; Blue/Roquefort salad dressing; Hoisin sauce; Table salt; Hot dog; Sofrito sauce; Table sugar (white or powder); various sauces; French salad dressing; Italian salad dressing; Nachos; Pizza; Chicken Nuggets; Capers; Breaded shrimp; Ketchup; Tabasco sauce; Mayonnaise; Fish sauce; Onion rings; Soy sauce; Hash brown potatoes; Horseradish; Macaroni; Tapioca; Syrup (table blends); Nutmeg (avoid only if it bothers you); Cheeseburger; Pickle relish; Gravies (canned);

Instead choose: Turmeric; Teriyaki sauce; Cardamom; Mints; Sweet pickle; Cloves; Falafel; Corn salad; Mace; Saffron; Fish stock; Corn cakes; Chives; Ginger; Licorice; Marjoram; Brown sugar; Vinegar; Clam chowder; Egg rolls (veg); Minestrone soup; Hamburger;

Alternative Therapies & Miscellaneous

2+ alcoholic drinks/day; Smoking, tobacco; Stress; Aspirin (& other NSAID drugs); Excess body weight; Fasting (for a specific period); Prescription drugs (NSAID containing drugs in particular); Food allergens (could cause problems for ulcer); Hyperthermia (avoid if extremely high blood pressure); Fried or battered foods; Processed or Refined foods; Salted foods, nuts, etc.; Corn sweetener; Fruit juice, sugared/concentrate;

Key Nutrients & Herbal Meds

Caffeine; Alcohol; Buckthorn (Herb); Saturated fat; Sodium (salt); Guarana; Kola (cola); Mate;

High Cholesterol & Ulcers

Cholesterol is a fat-like substance found in every cell of your body. Your body needs cholesterol to function properly, and it normally produces the amount of cholesterol that it requires. However, many foods that you consume can also result in increase in the level of cholesterol in your body -- in your blood in particular. There is usually no symptom for high cholesterol, but it can be discovered through a routine blood test.

High levels of cholesterol in your blood can result in build-up of what is known as plaque in your arteries. Plaque can narrow or block your arteries. Since arteries carry blood from your heart to the rest of your body, high level of cholesterol can result in heart disease and damage your cardiovascular system.

Cholesterol exists in two forms in your blood known as: LDL and HDL. LDL is called bad cholesterol because it leads to build up of plaque in your arteries. HDL is called good cholesterol because it removes and carries cholesterol away and delivers it to your liver where it gets eliminated from your body.

Your LDL is considered too high if it is greater than 160 milligram per deciliter. Your HDL is considered too low if it is less than 40 mg/dl. Your total cholesterol is considered too high if it is greater than 240 mg/dl, and is considered desirable if it is less than 200 mg/dl.

You are likely to have high cholesterol if you consume too much animal fat and trans fatty acids, you are not physically active, you are overweight, and there is a history of the same in your family. Your cholesterol levels tend to rise as you get older.

Choose these for High Cholesterol & Ulcers

Top 5 items to choose:

**Cabbage/Green leafy vegetables; Whole grains;
Kiwi fruit/Blackberries/Passion fruit; Dried Fruits;
Sun-dried tomatoes;**

Food items and actions that could improve your health (within a food group, most helpful items are listed first):

Meat, Fish & Poultry

Anchovy; Sardines; White fish; Marlin; Swordfish; Freshwater bass; Bluefish; Cisco (smoked); Drum; Halibut; Ling; King mackerel; Milkfish; Monkfish; Scup; Shark; Spot; Sturgeon; Sucker; Surimi; Tilapia; Tilefish; Trout; various tuna; Whiting; Wolffish; Yellowtail; Striped bass; Pollock; Snapper; Smelt; Carp; Seabass; White fish (smoked); Cusk; Flatfish (flounder & sole); Pout; Shad; Cisco; Northern pike; Mullet; Butterfish; Sablefish; Mussels; Lingcod; Rockfish; Seatrout; Haddock; Cod; Walleye; Grouper; Croaker; Catfish; Sheepshead; Turbot; Fish roe; Pumpkinseed sunfish; Salmon (smoked, Lox); Pink salmon; Dolphinfish (Mahi-Mahi); Herring; Perch; Pompano fish; Alaskan king crab; Clams; Burbot; Mackerel; Spiny lobster; Oysters; Chicken breast (no skin); Orange roughy; Dungeness crab; Caviar; Pheasant breast; Scallops; Beef filet mignon; Pork cured/ham; Pheasant; Veal loin; Chicken liver; Abalone;

Eggs, Beans, Nuts and Seeds

Soy milk; Split peas; Chia seeds; Fava beans; Sunflower seeds; Soybeans (green); Breadnut tree seeds; Beans: black, navy, yellow & white; Chickpeas; Lentils; various beans; Black-eyed peas; Sugar or snap peas; Soybean seeds; Lupin; Black walnuts; Ginkgo nuts; Pine nuts; Pistachio nuts; Safflower seeds; Hazelnuts or Filberts; Green peas; Sesame seeds; Flaxseed; Almonds[1]; Breadfruit seeds; Beechnuts; Walnuts; Cornnuts; Alfalfa sprouts; Peanuts; Pecans; Acorns; Hickory nuts; Butternuts; Pumpkin & squash seeds; Chestnuts; Egg white;

Fruits & Juices

Prunes (dried); Kiwi fruit; Dried pears; Blackberries; Dried figs; Passion fruit; Dried peaches; Avocado; Dried apples; Dried banana; Dried apricots; Abiyuch; Boysenberries; Currants (dried); Dates; various berries; Guava; Kumquats; Rowal; Tamarind; Raisins; Rhubarb; Dried fruits; Olives; Cranberries; Currants (raw); Goji berry; Cantaloupe; Plum; Apricots; Mango; Plantains; Pomegranate; Peaches; Grapes; Papaya; Breadfruit; Figs; Acerola; Cranberry juice; Jujube (fruit); Litchi; Longans; Persimmons; Durian; Pineapple; Pineapple juice; Cherries; Watermelon; Natal Plum (Carissa); Nectarine; Pomegranate juice; Banana; Strawberries; Grape juice; Prune juice; Pitanga; Honeydew melon; Quince; Blueberries; Pears; Apples (eat with skin); Apple juice (use fresh apples with skin); Lemon; Grapefruit; Lime; Pumelo (Shaddock); Grapefruit juice; Tangerines;

Vegetables

Grape leaves; Shitake mushrooms; Sun-dried tomatoes; Pigeon peas; Sweet potatoes leaves; Red cabbage (juice in particular); Dandelion Greens; Beet greens; Chicory greens; Collards; Mustard greens; Taro leaves; Turnip greens; Chinese broccoli; Savoy cabbage; Endive; Fungi cloud ears; Ancho peppers; Pasilla peppers; Chrysanthemum (Garland); Green cabbage (juice in particular); Spinach; Swiss chard; Garden cress; Kale; Pokeberry shoots; Watercress; Green onions (scallions); Bok choy; Wasabi root; Arugula; Jalapeno peppers; Balsam pear leafy tips; Romaine & loose leaf lettuce; Carrots; Amaranth leaves; Okra; Balsam pear; Kohlrabi; Sweet potatoes; Mustard spinach; various peppers; Asparagus; Winged beans leaves; Parsnips; Cauliflower; Garlic; Broccoli (sprouts in particular); Brussels sprouts; Green beans; Kelp; Portabella mushrooms; Pumpkin; Sesbania Flower; Tahitian taro; Tomato juice; Tomatoes; Vine spinach (Basella); Lotus root; Winter squash; Taro; Borage; Chrysanthemum Leaves; Cowpeas leafy tips; Fennel; Quinoa seed; Shallots; Yam; Epazote; Onions; Head lettuce; Fiddlehead ferns; Jew's ear mushrooms; Pumpkin flowers; Rutabaga; Purslane; Radishes; Artichoke; other vegetables;

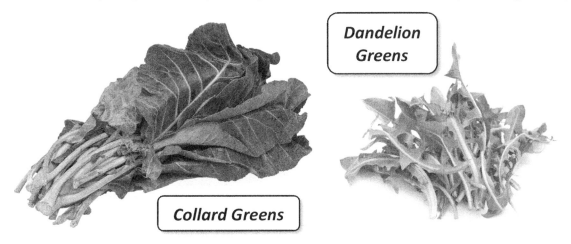

Dandelion Greens

Collard Greens

Breads, Grains, Cereals, Pasta

Rye; Corn bran; Durum wheat; Whole-wheat; Whole-wheat bread; Whole-wheat English muffins; Wheat germ; Whole-wheat cereal; Wheat germ cereal; Barley; Sorghum; Bran flakes cereal; Wheat bran muffins; Whole-wheat spaghetti; Whole-wheat crackers; Spelt (cooked); Bulgur; Rice bran; Oatmeal (cereal); Buckwheat; Triticale; Corn; Whole-wheat dinner rolls; Amaranth; Millet; Brown rice; Wild rice; Oat bran (3 grams per day for high cholesterol); Wheat bran; Chinese chow Mein noodles; Rice cakes (Brown rice based); Wheat germ bread; Bread sticks; Toasted bread; Pumpernickel bread; Oats; Oat bran bread; Corn flakes; Shredded wheat; Tortillas (corn); Semolina; Italian bread; Granola cereal; Oat bran muffins; English muffins; Corn muffins; Rice crisps cereal;

Dairy Products, Fats & Oils

Wheat Germ Oil; Yogurt; Olive oil; Canola oil; Whey (dried); Flaxseed oil; Fat-free or low fat products;

Desserts, Snacks, Beverages

Air-popped Popcorn; Oil popped popcorn; Sesame crunch candies; Peanut bar candy; Peanut butter; Honey (Manuka honey in particular); Potato chips/fried snacks; Water; Pumpkin pie; Fried pies (fruit);

Herbs & Spices, Prepared & Fast Foods

Cornmeal, whole-grain; Whole-grain Cornmeal; Parsley; Thyme (fresh); Tempeh; Tofu; Fried tofu; Miso; Coriander/Cilantro; Tomato paste; Rosemary (fresh); Peppermint; Mace; Croutons; Turmeric; Basil (fresh); Poppy seed; Natto; Egg rolls (veg); Cayenne (red) pepper; Cinnamon (for stomach ulcer in particular); Ginger; Malt syrup; Cole slaw; French fries; Mustard seed (avoid if it bothers you); Cloves; Clam chowder; Dill weed; Teriyaki sauce; Spearmint (fresh); Sage; Hummus; Corn cakes; Oregano; Mustard; Sweet pickle; Sauerkraut; Saffron; Succotash; Minestrone soup; Vegetable soup;

Alternative Therapies & Miscellaneous

Consult your doctor (check for H. Pylori); Exercise; Antacids; Elimination diet (to determine which foods cause problems for you); Glucomannan;

Key Nutrients & Herbal Medicines

Fiber (especially soluble fiber for ulcer); Psyllium; Slippery Elm (for stomach ulcer in particular); Fenugreek seeds; Celery seed; Monounsaturated fat (limit to 20% of total daily calories); Licorice (use in paste forms); Omega-3 fatty acids; Vitamin B-3 (Niacin in Nicotinic acid form); Yucca;

Do not choose these for High Cholesterol & Ulcers

Top 5 items to avoid:

Chocolate; Cheese; Cream & Butter; Luncheon (Processed) meats; Smoking;

Avoid or consume much less of the following (within a food group, most harmful items are listed first):

Meat, Fish & Poultry

Blood sausage; Pepperoni; Beef and pork frankfurter; Beef & pork luncheon meats; Chorizo; various sausage; Pastrami; Beerwurst beer salami; Bologna; Pork skins; Beef/Lamb tongue; Pork liver cheese; Chicken & turkey frankfurter; Pork ribs; Cured beef; Beef chuck/brisket; Pork spare ribs; various salami; Pork lungs; Beef jerky sticks; Lamb brain; Poultry skins; Organ meats; Lamb ribs; Squab (pigeon); Pork; Beef ribs; Cured meats; Ground lamb; Goose; Lamb; Beef shank; Bacon; Ground beef; Turkey dark meat; Bison/buffalo meat; Chicken dark meat; Shrimp;

Instead *choose:* *Veal shank; Octopus; Quail breast; Beef liver; Snail; Meatless sausage; Turkey liver; Guinea hen; Blue crab; Cured dried beef; Veal shoulder/leg/sirloin; Quail; Beef rib eye; Pork loin/sirloin; Veal liver; Cuttlefish; Beef round steak;*

Eggs, Beans, Nuts and Seeds

Coconut milk; Egg; Coconut; Egg substitute; Egg yolk; Pili nuts; Coconut meat (dried);

Instead *choose:* *Watermelon seeds; Cottonseed; Cashew nuts; Brazil nuts; Macadamia nuts;*

Breads, Grains, Cereals, Pasta

Croissant; Danish pastry; Sweet rolls; Donuts; Milk crackers; Saltines crackers; Cream of wheat; Waffles;

Instead choose: Biscuits; Wheat; Bagels; White rice; Spinach spaghetti; Banana bread; Melba toast crackers; Blueberry muffins; Couscous; various noodles; Spaghetti; Wheat crackers; White bread;

Dairy Products, Fats & Oils

Chocolate milk; Cream cheese; Goat cheese; Cream; Whipped cream; Cheese: Gjetost, Limburger, Roquefort; Butter; Cheese spread; various cheese; Sour cream; Lard; Animal fat; Poultry fat; Ucuhuba Butter oil; Hydrogenated vegetable oil; Cupu Assu oil; Babassu oil; Vegetable shortening; Oils: coconut, Shea nut, Cocoa Butter; Milk (determine if milk causes ulcer issues); Margarine-like spreads; Skim milk; various seeds/nuts/vegetable oils; various milk; Margarine (use soft or liquid vegetable-based oil based, if you must); Sardine fish oil; Menhaden fish oil; Sunflower oil;

Instead choose: Walnut oil; Safflower oil; Salmon fish oil; Hazelnut oil; Apricot kernel oil; Soybean oil;

Desserts, Snacks, Beverages

Chocolate ice cream; Sweet chocolate; Chocolate mousse; Dark chocolate; Pound cake; Butter cookies; Dessert toppings; Chocolate cake; Hot chocolate; Sponge cake; Éclairs; Lady fingers cookies; Cream puffs; Carob candy; Vanilla ice cream; After-dinner mints; Puff pastry; various cakes; Cheesecake; Coffee liqueur; various cookies; Pudding; Vanilla cream pie; 80+ proof distilled alcoholic beverages; Whiskey; Chocolate; Coffee; Crème de menthe; Coconut cream pie; Fruit leather/rolls; Piña colada; White wine; Eggnog; Frozen yogurt; Milk shakes; Taro chips; Lemon meringue pie; Coffeecake; Beer;

Instead **choose***: Tortilla chips; Green tea (do not brew or drink tea scolding hot); Peanut brittle; Halvah; Ice cream cones; Molasses; Frostings; Applesauce; Fruit punch; Ginger ale; Sports drinks; Herbal tea; Plain tea (avoid if it bothers you); Tonic water;*

Herbs & Spices. Prepared & Fast Foods

Chocolate syrup; Cheese sauce; Nachos; Foie gras or liver pate; Hot dog; Pizza; Chicken Nuggets; Blue/Roquefort salad dressing; Table sugar (white or powder); Breaded shrimp; Macaroni; Barbecue sauce; Tapioca sauce; Cheeseburger; Oyster sauce; Tabasco sauce; Ketchup; Sofrito sauce; Hush puppies; French toast; Fish sauce; Hoisin sauce; French salad dressing; Nutmeg; Italian salad dressing;

Instead **choose***: Cottonseed meal; Fish stock; Corn salad; Tarragon (dried); Fennel seeds; Pickle relish; Hash brown potatoes; Cardamom; Mayonnaise; Veg/beef soup; Chives; Pickle (cucumber);*

Alternative Therapies & Miscellaneous

Smoking, tobacco; 2+ alcoholic drinks/day; Fried or battered foods; Aspirin (& other NSAID containing drugs); Fasting (for a specific period); Prescription drugs; Baking using butter; Processed or Refined foods; Excess body weight; Food allergens (need to determine which foods cause problems for Ulcers); Stress;

Key Nutrients & Herbal Medicines

Saturated fat (limit to 7% of daily calories); Cholesterol (less than 200 mg per day); Alcohol; Buckthorn (Herb); Caffeine; Trans fatty acids;

Menopause & Ulcers

Elderly women (over 60 years old) who regularly take NSAIDs or other pain medications for osteoarthritis or other health issues are at a high risk to develop Peptic ulcers. It is for that reason that we are including this chapter on nutrition considerations for menopausal women with Ulcers.

Menopause is the time in a woman's life when she has not had a period for over a year. All women experience menopause and on average at the age of 51 years old. Menopause is triggered when the ovaries stop producing certain hormones (estrogen and progesterone) either naturally or due to certain medical treatments or surgeries.

Menopause and change in hormone levels in a woman's body happen over time and can result in a number of symptoms. Most common symptom is hot flashes (also called hot flushes) which is a sudden feeling of heat and sweating in face, neck and upper body that can last as long as ten minutes. Other common symptoms include: sleeping difficulties, vaginal dryness, urinary problems, mood swings, change of attitude or interest in sex, forgetfulness, and inability to focus.

Changes in your body during this period can result in certain health issues including greater risk of heart disease, stroke and osteoporosis. A balanced diet; adequate intake of calcium, iron and Vitamin D; exercise; quitting smoking; and regular check-ups are all important considerations to your health and coping with menopause symptoms.

Choose these for Ulcers & Menopause

Top 5 items to choose:

Green leafy vegetables; Prunes & Raisins; Whole Grains; Pine nuts; Soy milk;

Food items and actions that could improve your health (within a food group, most helpful items are listed first):

Meat, Fish & Poultry

Oysters; Snail; Spiny lobster; Carp; Sardines; White fish; Fish roe; Marlin; Swordfish; Salmon (smoked, Lox); Pink salmon; Snapper; Bear meat; Catfish; Sturgeon; Trout;

Eggs, Beans, Nuts and Seeds

Pine nuts; Soy milk; Split peas; Chia seeds; Almonds; Sunflower seeds; Soybeans (green); Hazelnuts or Filberts; Soybean seeds; Peanuts; Fava beans; Safflower seeds; Hyacinth beans; Black beans; Navy beans; Lentils; Green peas; Winged beans; Watermelon seeds; Alfalfa sprouts; various beans; Black walnuts; Cottonseed; Cashew nuts; various beans; Flaxseed; Pistachio nuts; Brazil nuts; Sugar or snap peas; Pecans; Lupin; Breadnut tree seeds; Black-eyed peas; Sesame seeds; Butternuts; Pumpkin & squash seeds; Chickpeas; Hickory nuts; Lima beans; Walnuts; Breadfruit seeds;

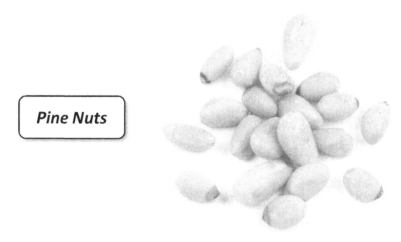

Pine Nuts

Fruits & Juices

Prunes (dried); Raisins; Dried fruits: figs, banana, peaches, pears; Passion fruit; dried apricots; Avocado; Tamarind; Grape juice; Dates; Blackberries; dried apples; Kiwi fruit; Currants (dried); dried fruits; Cranberry juice; Prune juice; Plantains; Abiyuch; Boysenberries; various berries; Guava; Kumquats; Rowal; Pears; Apple juice; Pomegranate; Pineapple juice; Pomegranate juice; Breadfruit; Currants (raw); Durian; Figs; Grapes; Goji berry; Blueberries; Apples; Peaches; Acerola; Apricots; Cantaloupe; Cherries; Cowberries; Honeydew melon; Jujube (fruit); Litchi; Longans; Mango; Natal Plum (Carissa); Nectarine; Papaya; Persimmons; Pineapple; Pitanga; Plum; Quince; Strawberries; Watermelon; Banana; Rhubarb; Cranberries; Olives; Grapefruit juice; Orange juice;

Vegetables

Grape leaves; Shitake mushrooms; Pigeon peas; Sun-dried tomatoes; Fungi cloud ears; Pasilla & ancho peppers; Dandelion Greens; Collards; Taro leaves; Kelp; Sweet potatoes leaves; Wasabi root; Chicory greens; Mustard greens; Turnip greens; Amaranth leaves; Epazote; Chinese broccoli; Chrysanthemum (Garland); Kale; Arugula; Green cabbage (juice in particular); Artichoke; Balsam pear leafy tips; Watercress; Savoy cabbage; Endive; Green onions (scallions); Red cabbage (juice in particular); Garden cress; Asparagus; Bok choy; Romaine & loose leaf lettuce; Okra; Pokeberry shoots; Mustard spinach; Jalapeno peppers; Winged beans leaves; Beet greens; Parsnips; Chrysanthemum Leaves; Leeks; Taro; Quinoa seed; Spinach; Carrots; Green beans; Nopal; Tahitian taro; Vine spinach (Basella); Potatoes w/skin; Lotus root; Cauliflower; Celery; Head lettuce; Balsam pear; Eggplant; Kohlrabi; Banana peppers; Shallots; Yam; Arrowhead; Swiss chard; Red bell peppers; Garlic; Borage; Cowpeas leafy tips; Cucumbers with peel; Purslane; Potato; Arrowroot; Jerusalem artichoke; Portabella mushrooms; other vegetables;

Breads, Grains, Cereals, Pasta

Wheat germ cereal; Wheat bran; Wheat germ; Buckwheat; Rye; Rice bran; Durum wheat; Amaranth; Whole-wheat; Corn bran; Oats; Whole-wheat bread; Triticale; Wheat germ bread; Whole-wheat cereal; Whole-wheat English muffins; Whole-wheat spaghetti; Oatmeal (cereal); Wheat bran muffins; Granola cereal; Spelt (cooked); Sorghum; Bran flakes cereal; Wild rice; Barley; Bulgur; Shredded wheat cereal; Millet; Brown rice; Corn; Oat bran; Tortillas (corn); Oat bran muffins; Rice cakes (Brown rice based); Whole-wheat crackers;

Dairy Products, Fats & Oils

Wheat Germ Oil; Yogurt; Canola oil;

Desserts, Snacks, Beverages

Air-popped Popcorn; Sesame crunch candies; Tonic water; Water; Sports drinks; Ginger ale; Honey (Manuka honey in particular); Peanut butter; Fruit punch; Lemonade; Molasses; Halvah; Peanut bar; Tortilla chips;

Herbs & Spices, Fast Foods, Prepared Foods

Tofu; Cottonseed meal; Thyme (fresh); Tempeh; Fried tofu; Whole-grain cornmeal; Rosemary (fresh); Natto; Peppermint; Parsley; Basil (fresh); Maple sugar; Cinnamon (for stomach ulcer in particular); Spearmint (fresh); Cayenne (red) pepper; Coriander/Cilantro; Oregano; Poppy seed; Cheese fondue; Sage; Cole slaw; French fries;

Alternative Therapies & Miscellaneous

Consult your doctor (test for H. Pylori); Salt-free or low-salt foods; Acupuncture; Antacids; Elimination diet (to determine which foods cause problems for Ulcers); Fluids/juices/water; Relaxation/breathing techniques (deep breathing to reduce hot flashes); Exposure to sun;

Key Nutrients & Herbal Medicines

Slippery Elm (for stomach ulcer in particular); Black cohosh; Calcium[7]; Corn silk (take in herbal tea form for its diuretic effect); Fiber; Licorice (in paste form for Ulcers); Zinc; Vitamin E (for menopause symptoms); Fenugreek seeds;

Do not choose these for Ulcers & Menopause

Top 5 items to avoid:

Chocolate & Sweets; Alcoholic beverages;
Luncheon (Processed) Meats; Coffee; &
Smoking/Tobacco;

Avoid or consume much less of the following (within a food group, most harmful items are listed first):

Meat, Fish & Poultry

Blood sausage; Pepperoni; Frankfurters; Chorizo; Luncheon (processed) meats; Sausage; Pastrami; Salami; Pork skins; Pork liver cheese; Bacon; Pork breakfast strips; Cured beef; Bologna; Cured meats; Beef jerky sticks; Caviar; Pork cured/ham; Poultry skins; Clams; Pork headcheese; Corned beef; Shrimp; Anchovy; Lamb tongue; White fish (smoked); Squab (pigeon); Croaker; Pork ribs; Beef tongue; Calamari; Cuttlefish; Lamb ribs; Veal lungs; Lamb brain; Veal spleen; Pork spare ribs; Sablefish; Chicken wings; Veal thymus; Haddock; Pork heart; Lamb loin; Goose;

Instead choose: Veal shank; Veal liver; Beef filet mignon; Perch; Lamb liver; Ground beef; Pork liver; Blue fin tuna; Seabass; Pumpkinseed sunfish; Dungeness crab; Chicken heart; Caribou meat; Beef round steak; Halibut; Pork loin/sirloin; Veal shoulder/leg/sirloin; Beef rib eye; Whelk; Herring; Octopus; Blue crab; Northern pike; Canned tuna; Lamb leg; Tilapia; Yellowfin tuna; Mackerel; Ling; Freshwater bass; Walleye; Eel; Pout; Rockfish; Quail breast; Surimi; Beef liver; Beef top sirloin; Mussels; Pompano fish; Shad; Smelt; Crayfish; Whiting; other fish;

Eggs, Beans, Nuts and Seeds

Coconut milk; Egg substitute; Egg;

Instead choose: Ginkgo nuts; Chestnuts; Pili nuts; Coconut meat (dried); Acorns; Beechnuts; Cornnuts; Egg white; Macadamia nuts;

Breads, Grains, Cereals, Pasta

Croissant; Saltines crackers; Danish pastry; Rice crisps cereal; Sweet rolls; Kaiser dinner rolls; French rolls; Milk crackers; Wheat crackers; Donuts; Hamburger & hot dog rolls; Biscuits; Corn flakes; Waffles; Melba toasts; Bagels; Bread sticks; White bread;

Instead choose: Pumpernickel bread; Whole-wheat dinner rolls; Toasted bread; Corn muffins; Semolina; Oat bran bread; White rice; Wheat; Spinach spaghetti; various noodles; Couscous; Spaghetti; Cornbread;

Dairy Products, Fats & Oils

Chocolate milk; Roquefort cheese; Butter (salted); Pimento cheese; Brie cheese; Cheese spread; various cheese; Butter (unsalted); Whipped cream; Lard; Animal fat; Cream; Oils: sesame, coconut, Cupu Assu, Shea nut, tea seed, Ucuhuba Butter; Poultry fat; Sour cream; Margarine (salted); Hydrogenated vegetable oil; Sardine fish oil; Menhaden fish oil; Milk (determine if problem for Ulcers); Walnut oil; Flaxseed oil; various fish oil; Margarine-like spreads; Skim milk; Whey (dried);

Instead **choose**: *Hazelnut oil; Safflower oil; Cottage cheese; Margarine (unsalted); Oil, olive; Almonds oil; Grape seeds oil; Cod liver fish oil; Soybean oil; Swiss cheese; Sunflower oil;*

Desserts, Snacks, Beverages

Coffee liqueur; Chocolate ice cream; Sweet chocolate; Dark chocolate; Pound cake; Butter cookies; 80+ proof distilled alcoholic beverages; Whiskey; Chocolate chip cookies; Coffee (to avoid hot flashes); various cookies; Chocolate mousse; Crème de menthe; various cakes; Éclairs; Cream puffs; Pretzels; Pie crust; Piña colada; Puff pastry; Cheesecake; Dessert toppings; Fruit leather/rolls; Vanilla cream pie; Coffeecake; Hot chocolate; Vanilla ice cream; Red wine; White wine; After-dinner mints; Pudding; Potato sticks; Plain tea; various pies; Ice cream cones; Pancakes; Beer; Green tea;

Instead **choose**: *Oil popped popcorn; Carob candies; Jellies; Applesauce; Herbal tea; Malted drinks (nonalcoholic); Potato chips; Hard candies; Marshmallows;*

Herbs & Spices, Fast Foods, Prepared Foods

Foie gras or liver pate; Barbecue sauce; Fish sauce; Oyster sauce; various sauces; Hot dog; Blue/Roquefort salad dressing; Capers; Table salt; Ketchup; Nachos; Italian salad dressing; Chicken Nuggets; Breaded shrimp; Chocolate syrup; Tabasco sauce; Potato pancakes; Table sugar (white or powder); Pizza; French salad dressing; Cocoa; Mustard; Potato salad; Hash brown potatoes; Pickle relish; Hush puppies; Horseradish; Soy sauce; French toast; Macaroni; Tapioca; Onion rings; Gravies (canned); Mayonnaise; Nutmeg (avoid only if bothers you); Pickle (cucumber); Cheeseburger; Beef broth; Veg/beef soup; Egg rolls (veg);

Instead **choose**: *Chervil; Cardamom; Dill weed; Fennel seeds; Mints; Succotash; Tarragon; Cloves; Mace; Turmeric; Sweet pickle; Miso; Maple & Sorghum syrups; Chives; Ginger; Marjoram; Saffron; Brown sugar; Vinegar; Hamburger; Malt syrup;*

Alternative Therapies & Miscellaneous

Smoking, tobacco (also to avoid hot flashes); Alcoholic beverages; Aspirin (& other NSAID containing drugs); Fasting (for a specific period); Spicy foods (does not cause Ulcers but can worsen symptoms; avoiding also helps to avoid hot flashes); Prescription drugs; Stress; Salted foods, nuts, etc.; Food allergens (determine if a food causes problems for Ulcers); Very hot drinks/soups (to avoid hot flashes); Processed or Refined foods; Fried or battered foods; Baking using butter;

Key Nutrients & Herbal Medicines

Alcohol (avoidance also helps with hot flashes); Caffeine; Sodium (salt); Buckthorn (Herb); Saturated fat; Guarana; Kola (cola); Mate;

Stress & Ulcers

Everyone experiences some sort of stress almost every day. Stress is our brain's response to a demand. Not everyone reacts to the same events or demands the same way. What may be stressful to one person may not be to another. It is stress that drives us to act, and in some cases such as survival situations, perform beyond our normal abilities. However, long term or chronic stress can lead to a variety of problems including illnesses such as high blood pressure, depression and cancer.

Chronic stress can be caused by a number of factors, among them: bad childhood experiences (whose pain and impact you have never been able to escape), poverty and helplessness, an unhappy marriage, never-ending tension and violence all around you, a wrong job or career, and a dysfunctional family.

Chronic stress challenges our mind and body over a long time, and thus may require an on-going treatment over an extended period of time.

While stress can worsen your ulcer symptoms, it is not a cause for ulcers.

Choose these for   Ulcers & Stress

Top 5 items to choose:

Red & Green cabbage; Green Leafy
Vegetables; Kiwi fruit/Guava; Sun-dried
tomatoes; Jalapeno & other peppers;

Food items and actions that could improve your health (within a food group, most helpful items are listed first):

Meat, Fish & Poultry

Liver; Spleen; Yellowfin tuna; Veal thymus; Whelk; Octopus; Beef filet mignon; Veal lungs; Pancreas (lamb, beef, veal); Marlin; Swordfish; Turkey & Chicken heart; Alaskan King crab; Spiny lobster; Pink salmon; Clams; Turkey giblets; Beef rib eye; Beef top sirloin; Halibut; Fish roe; Cured dried beef; Beef round steak; Veal shank; Beef; Dungeness crab; Bluefish; King mackerel; Milkfish; Snapper; Spot; Blue fin tuna; Wolffish; Oysters; Blue crab; Heart; Cusk; Cuttlefish; Kidneys; Rabbit meat; Pollock; Veal shoulder/leg/sirloin; Pheasant; Bison/buffalo meat; Striped bass; Drum; Shark; Sheepshead; Mackerel; Caviar; Butterfish; Haddock; Lingcod; Scup; Seatrout; Tilefish; White fish (smoked); Herring; Chicken breast (no skin); Sardines; Shrimp; Quail; Veal loin; Lamb leg; Veal tongue; Pork loin/sirloin; White fish; Carp; Smelt; Perch; Pumpkinseed sunfish; Meatless sausage; Corned beef; Mussels; Lobster; Dolphinfish (Mahi-Mahi); Sturgeon; Sucker; Turbot; Cisco; Rockfish; Salmon (smoked, Lox); Trout; Whiting; Abalone; Sablefish; Freshwater bass; Northern pike; Walleye; Surimi; Catfish; Tilapia; Canned tuna; Anchovy; Crayfish; Bologna; Scallops; Seabass; Burbot; Yellowtail; Pout; Mullet; Brain; Shad; Lamb; Croaker; Flatfish (flounder & sole); Boar meat; Turkey breast; Beef jerky sticks; Ling; Pork cured/ham; Salami; Tongue; Snail; Cod; Grouper; Calamari; Monkfish; Eel; Turkey dark meat; Pork back ribs; Chorizo; Bacon; Pompano fish; Guinea hen;

Eggs, Beans, Nuts and Seeds

Breadnut tree seeds; Sunflower seeds; Sugar or snap peas; Safflower seeds; Green peas; Ginkgo nuts; Soy milk; Pistachio nuts; Flaxseed; Pine nuts; Cottonseed; Hazelnuts or Filberts; Chestnuts; Sesame seeds; Soybean seeds; Split peas; Beechnuts; Black walnuts; Soybeans (green); Almonds; Chia seeds; Butternuts; Peanuts; Acorns; Cashew nuts; Watermelon seeds; Walnuts; Egg yolk; Pumpkin & squash seeds; Duck & goose eggs; Fava beans; Lentils; Pecans; Breadfruit seeds; Egg substitute; Pinto beans; Boiled & poached egg; Coconut meat (dried); Yardlong beans; Alfalfa sprouts; Hickory nuts; Cornnuts; Brazil nuts;

Fruits & Juices

Kiwi fruit; Abiyuch; Guava; Currants (raw); Dried litchi; Acerola; Jujube (fruit); Litchi; Longans; Papaya; Persimmons; Pineapple juice; Strawberries; Kumquats; Prunes (dried); Elderberries; Dried banana; Pineapple; Currants (dried); Goji berry; Passion fruit; Avocado; Dried pears; Cantaloupe; Mango; Mulberries; Natal Plum (Carissa); Dates; Dried fruits; Lemon; Raisins; Plantains; Tamarind; Blackberries; Breadfruit; Boysenberries; Pomegranate; Prune juice; Rhubarb; Banana; Olives; Berries; Cranberries; Figs; Grapes; Pears; Pomegranate juice; Rowal; Durian; Apple juice; Apples; Apricots; Cherries; Cranberry juice; Grape juice; Nectarine; Peaches; Plum; Watermelon; Pitanga; Orange juice; Oranges; Pumelo (Shaddock); Honeydew melon; Quince; Grapefruit juice;

Vegetables

Sun-dried tomatoes; Red cabbage (juice in particular for Ulcers); Mustard greens; Taro leaves; Turnip greens; Balsam pear leafy tips; Garden cress; Kale; Pokeberry shoots; Amaranth leaves; Shitake mushrooms; Dandelion Greens; Wasabi root; Collards; Watercress; Bok choy; Green cabbage (juice in particular); Peppers: jalapeno, ancho, pasilla; Balsam pear; Kohlrabi; Mustard spinach; Banana pepper; Broccoli (sprouts in particular); Red bell peppers; Spinach; Savoy cabbage; Cauliflower; Winged beans leaves; Green bell peppers; Hot chili peppers; Pimento peppers; Sesbania Flower; Tahitian taro; Vine spinach (Basella); Beet greens; Lambsquarters; Swiss chard; Chinese broccoli; Brussels sprouts; Garlic; Cowpeas leafy tips; Grape leaves; Chicory greens; Borage; Okra; Pigeon peas; Sweet potatoes leaves; Green onions (scallions); Fungi cloud ears; Arugula; Lotus root; Pumpkin flowers; Chrysanthemum (Garland); Kelp; Endive; Purslane; Romaine or loose leaf lettuce; Sweet potatoes; Parsnips; Rutabaga; Leeks; Asparagus; Yellow squash; Zucchini; Shallots; other vegetables;

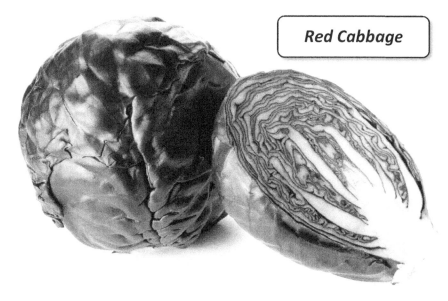

Red Cabbage

Breads, Grains, Cereals, Pasta

Wheat bran; Wheat germ cereal; Wheat germ; Bran flakes cereal; Rice bran; Wheat bran muffins; Amaranth; Wheat germ bread; Durum wheat; Whole-wheat; Rye; Buckwheat; Corn bran; Corn flakes; Rice crisps cereal; Shredded wheat cereal; Whole-wheat spaghetti; Whole-wheat cereal; Whole-wheat bread; Whole-wheat English muffins; Triticale; Whole-wheat crackers; Oatmeal (cereal); Spelt (cooked); Brown rice; Sorghum; Whole-wheat dinner rolls; Barley; Bulgur; Wild rice; Millet; Corn; Oats; Granola cereal; Oat bran muffins; Oat bran; Rice cakes (Brown rice based); Tortillas (corn);

Dairy Products, Fats & Oils

Wheat germ oil; Whey (dried); Yogurt; Canola oil;

Desserts, Snacks, Beverages

Air-popped popcorn; Potato sticks; Fruit leather/rolls; Potato chips; Sesame crunch candies; Honey (Manuka honey in particular); Oil popped popcorn; Molasses; Peanut butter; Halvah; Tortilla chips; Peanut bar;

Herbs & Spices, Fast Foods, Prepared Foods

Parsley; Thyme (fresh); Cottonseed meal; Dill weed; Whole-grain cornmeal; Rosemary (fresh); Cole slaw; Coriander/Cilantro; Corn salad; Peppermint; Potato pancakes; Basil (fresh); Tofu; Tomato paste; Cayenne (red) pepper; Sorghum syrup; Sofrito sauce; Tempeh; Miso; Teriyaki sauce; Natto; Malt syrup; Clam chowder; Cinnamon (for stomach ulcer in particular); Fried tofu; French fries; Tarragon (dried); Spearmint (fresh); Hummus; Sauerkraut; Maple sugar; Oregano;

Alternative Therapies & Miscellaneous

Consult your doctor (check for H. Pylori); Antacids; Biofeedback; Elimination diet (to determine problem foods); Exercise regularly; Laugh, laughter; Meditation; Sexual activity; Sleep 6-8 hours regularly; Take a vacation!; Yoga;

Key Nutrients & Herbal Medicines

Slippery Elm (for stomach ulcer in particular); Vitamin C; Ashwaganda; Asian & Siberian Ginseng; Licorice (use in past form for Ulcers); Vitamin B-6;

<u>*Do not*</u> choose these for   Ulcers & Stress

Top 5 items to avoid:

Chocolate; Aspirin & other drugs; Coffee; Alcoholic Beverages; Fasting; & Smoking;

Avoid or consume much less of the following (within a food group, most harmful items are listed first):

Meat, Fish & Poultry

There are no items in this food group that could worsen your conditions.

Instead <u>choose</u>: Chicken dark meat; Pork; Goose; Duck (no skin); Chicken wings; Orange roughy; Venison; Chicken & turkey frankfurters; Squab (pigeon); Pepperoni;

Eggs, Beans, Nuts and Seeds

Coconut Milk;

Instead <u>choose</u>: Raw egg; various beans; Chickpeas; Black-eyed peas; Macadamia nuts; Lupin; Pili nuts; Egg white; Coconut;

Breads, Grains, Cereals, Pasta

Croissant;

Instead <u>choose</u>: Toasted bread; Pumpernickel bread; Wheat crackers; Chinese chow Mein noodles; Banana bread; Oat bran bread; Semolina. Bread sticks; Italian bread; English muffins; Corn muffins; Wheat; Cream of wheat; Granola bars; Melba toasts; Cornbread; Spaghetti spinach; Bagels; Couscous; Blueberry muffins; various noodles; Pasta; White rice; Spaghetti; Waffles; Matzo crackers;

Dairy Products, Fats & Oils

Chocolate milk; Milk (determine if it causes problems for your Ulcers); Cream; Whipped cream; Butter; Goat cheese; Cream cheese; Sour cream; Lard; Animal fat; Roquefort cheese; Skim milk; Sesame oil; Pimento cheese; Oils: coconut, Cupu Assu, Shea nut, tea seed, Ucuhuba Butter; Ricotta cheese;

Instead <u>choose</u>: Margarine; Olive oil; Soybean oil; Feta cheese; Margarine-like spreads; Hazelnut & Safflower oils; various cheese; Vegetable shortening; Almonds oil; Grape seeds oil; Apricot kernel oil;

Desserts, Snacks, Beverages

Coffee liqueur; Sweet chocolate; Dark chocolate; Chocolate ice cream; Hot chocolate; Coffee; 80+ proof distilled alcoholic beverages; Whiskey; Crème de menthe; Piña colada; Red wine; White wine; Chocolate chip cookies; Chocolate mousse; Plain tea; Pound cake; various cookies; Beer; Dessert toppings; Chocolate cake; Vanilla ice cream;

Instead <u>choose</u>: Taro chips; Water; Caramel candies; Pumpkin pie; various candies; Frostings; Applesauce; Fruit punch; Ginger ale; Lemonade; Sports drinks; Herbal tea; Tonic water; Pecan pie; Eggnog; Malted (nonalcoholic) drinks; Carob candies; Pretzels;

Herbs & Spices, Fast Foods, Prepared Foods

Cocoa; Chocolate syrup; Cheese sauce; Nutmeg (avoid only if bothers you); Table sugar (white or powder); Mustard seed (avoid only if it bothers you);

Instead *choose*: *Fish sauce; Hamburger; Soy sauce; Sage; Sweet pickle; Chives; Cheeseburger; Cheese fondue; Chervil; Turmeric; Pickle (cucumber); Foie gras or liver pate; Poppy seed; Cloves; Taco shells; Fish stock; Beef broth; Beef stock; Chicken broth; Chicken noodle soup; Chicken stock; Veg/beef soup; Cardamom; Croutons; Mayonnaise; Saffron; French salad dressing; Corn cakes; Mustard; Succotash; Italian salad dressing; Breaded shrimp; Egg rolls (veg); Fennel seeds; Mace; Pickle relish; Maple syrup; Hash brown potatoes; Chicken nuggets; Falafel; Hush puppies; Nachos; Capers; Ginger; Gravies; Horseradish; Marjoram; Table salt; Brown sugar; Syrup (table blends); Vinegar; Pizza; French toast; Hot dog; Onion rings;*

Alternative Therapies & Miscellaneous

Prescription drugs (especially NSAID drugs); Alcoholic beverages; Aspirin (& other NSAID drugs); Fasting (for a specific period); Smoking, tobacco; Food allergens (need to avoid foods that cause problems for your Ulcers); Stress; FD&C yellow dye #5. Tartrazine;

Key Nutrients & Herbal Medicines

Caffeine; Alcohol; Buckthorn (Herb); Guarana; Kola (cola); Mate;

Vitamin D Deficiency & Ulcers

Vitamin D Deficiency is a common problem for many people especially the older people. Vitamin D is a critical nutrient for your body in particular for stronger bones, muscle movements, nerve function and immune system well-being.

You will develop this deficiency if you don't absorb enough Vitamin D from your diet, you don't get enough exposure to the sun (especially during the winter months), your skin cannot convert the sun exposure to Vitamin D (as in elderly and darker skin), or you are obese. You can also develop this deficiency if your body cannot properly process fats due to Celiac or Crohn's disease, since fats are required for Vitamin D absorption into your blood. Health issues with kidney and liver can also result in this deficiency because they can prevent your body to process Vitamin D.

Adults, ages 19 to 70, require 600 IU (International Units) of Vitamin D per day. Adults, ages 71 and above, require 800 IU per day.

Meeting your Vitamin D needs entirely through sun exposure or tanning is not recommended due to the risk of skin cancer. Too much Vitamin D in your blood (almost always caused by supplements) can also be harmful.

Choose these for Ulcers & Vitamin D Deficiency

Top 5 items to choose:

Fish Roe; Prunes; Fish; Catch some sun; Shitake mushrooms;

Food items and actions that could improve your health (within a food group, most helpful items are listed first):

Meat, Fish & Poultry

Fish roe; Carp; White fish; Marlin; Swordfish; Catfish; Cisco (smoked); Pink salmon; Snapper; Sturgeon; Trout; White fish (smoked); Eel; Mackerel; Pompano fish; Seabass; Halibut; Blue fin tuna; Herring; Sardines; Perch; Alaskan King crab; Flatfish (flounder & sole); Spiny lobster; Oysters; Rockfish; Shad; Tilapia; Anchovy; Pork liver;

Eggs, Beans, Nuts and Seeds

Split peas; Pine nuts; Soybean seeds; Almonds; Soy milk; Fava beans; Chia seeds; Hazelnuts or Filberts; Soybeans (green); Peanuts; Flaxseed; Green peas; Sunflower seeds; Alfalfa sprouts; Egg yolk; Beans: black, navy, yellow & white; Chickpeas; Lentils; Hyacinth beans; Pecans; Safflower seeds; Adzuki beans; Black-eyed peas; Mung beans; Pinto beans; Sugar or snap peas; Winged beans;

Fruits & Juices

Prunes (dried); Raisins; Avocado; Kiwi fruit; Dried pears; Blackberries; Dried figs; Passion fruit; Dried peaches; Plantains; Dates; Dried fruits; Pears; Abiyuch; Boysenberries; Currants (dried); various berries; Guava; Kumquats; Pomegranate; Rhubarb; Rowal; Tamarind; Grapes; Olives; Grape juice; Blueberries and Bilberries; Breadfruit; Cranberries; Currants (raw); Durian; Figs; Goji berry; Pomegranate juice; Apples; Peaches; Acerola; Apple juice; Apricots; Cantaloupe; Cherries; Cranberry juice; Honeydew melon; Jujube (fruit); Litchi; Longans; Mango; Natal Plum (Carissa); Nectarine; Papaya; Persimmons; Pineapple; Pineapple juice; Pitanga; Plum; Prune juice; Quince; Strawberries; Watermelon; Banana;

Vegetables

Shitake mushrooms; Grape leaves; Sun-dried tomatoes; Pigeon peas; Sweet potatoes leaves; Green & red cabbage (juice in particular); Dandelion Greens; Beet greens; Chicory greens; Collards; Mustard greens; Taro leaves; Turnip greens; Chinese broccoli; Savoy cabbage; Chrysanthemum (Garland); Endive; Fungi cloud ears; Green onions (scallions); Kelp; Ancho & pasilla peppers; Spinach; Swiss chard; Amaranth leaves; Arugula; Balsam pear leafy tips; Garden cress; Kale; Romaine & loose leaf lettuce; Pokeberry shoots; Watercress; Asparagus; Artichoke; Bok choy; Leeks; Okra; Wasabi root; Parsnips; Jalapeno peppers; Cauliflower; Carrots; Celery; Epazote; Green beans; Head lettuce; Taro; Balsam pear; Chrysanthemum Leaves; Cucumbers with peel; Eggplant; Fennel; Hearts of palm; Kohlrabi; Lotus root; Mustard spinach; various peppers; Quinoa seed; Shallots; Sweet potatoes; Winged beans leaves; Yam; Broccoli; Brussels sprouts; Garlic; Potato; Red bell peppers; other vegetables;

Breads, Grains, Cereals, Pasta

Rye; Corn bran; Durum wheat; Buckwheat; Whole-wheat; Bran flakes cereal; Amaranth; Wheat bran; Whole-wheat cereal; Wheat germ cereal; Whole-wheat bread; Whole-wheat English muffins; Triticale; Whole-wheat spaghetti; Wheat germ; Sorghum; Spelt (cooked); Wheat bran muffins; Barley; Bulgur; Rice bran; Wild rice; Whole-wheat crackers; Oatmeal (cereal); Corn; Millet; Brown rice; Wheat germ bread; Whole-wheat dinner rolls; Oat bran; Oats; Corn flakes;

Dairy Products, Fats & Oils

Cod liver fish oil; Yogurt; Wheat germ oil; Canola oil;

Desserts, Snacks, Beverages

Air popped popcorn; Honey (Manuka in particular); Oil popped popcorn;

Herbs & Spices, Fast Foods, Prepared Foods

Whole-grain cornmeal; Tofu; Coriander/Cilantro; Parsley; Basil (fresh); Cayenne (red) pepper; Cinnamon (for stomach ulcer in particular); Cole slaw; Cottonseed meal; Natto; Thyme (fresh); Tempeh; Maple sugar; Teriyaki sauce;

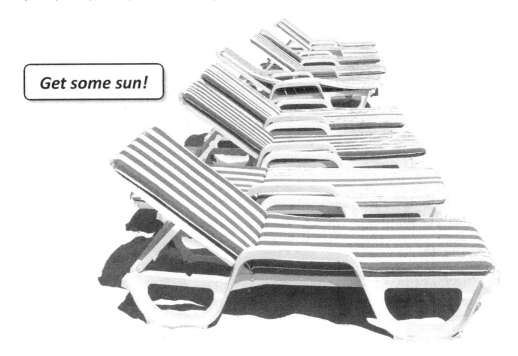

Get some sun!

Alternative Therapies & Miscellaneous

Consult your doctor (test for H. Pylori bacteria); Exposure to Sun (ten minutes per day); Antacids; Elimination diet (to determine which foods cause problems for your Ulcers);

Key Nutrients & Herbal Medicines

Slippery Elm (for stomach ulcer); Vitamin D; Licorice (in paste form for Ulcers);

Do not choose these for Ulcers & Vitamin D Deficiency

Top 5 items to avoid:

Chocolate; Aspirin & Prescription drugs; Fasting; Caffeine/Coffee/Cocoa; Alcoholic beverages;

Avoid or consume much less of the following (within a food group, most harmful items are listed first):

Meat, Fish & Poultry

Blood sausage; Pepperoni; Beef and pork sausage; Beef & pork luncheon meats; Liver sausage; Luncheon (processed) meats; various sausage; Turkey pastrami; various salami;

Instead choose: Chicken heart; Liver; Veal shank; Dungeness crab; Caviar; Abalone; Blue crab; Pork cured/ham; Pork loin/sirloin; Cuttlefish; Lobster; Mullet; Octopus; Northern pike; Walleye; Yellowfin tuna; Whiting; Cured dried beef; Beef filet mignon; Beef round steak; Veal shoulder/leg/sirloin; Beef; Pork; Snail; Clams; Mussels; Whelk; Kidneys; Spleen; Corned beef; Lamb heart; Lamb leg; Pancreas (lamb, beef, veal); Veal tongue; Crayfish; Shrimp;

Eggs, Beans, Nuts and Seeds

Coconut milk;

Instead choose: Breadnut tree seeds; Cashew nuts; Watermelon seeds; Baked beans; Kidney beans; Lupin; Black walnuts; Pistachio nuts; Moth beans; Yardlong beans; Sesame seeds; Pumpkin & squash seeds; Lima beans; Egg; Cottonseed; Cornnuts; Butternuts; Breadfruit seeds; Chestnuts; Hickory nuts; Ginkgo nuts;

Fruits & Juices

Lemon; Lime; Grapefruit; Grapefruit juice; Orange juice; Oranges; Pumelo (Shaddock); Tangerines;

Breads, Grains, Cereals, Pasta

Croissant;

Instead choose: Shredded wheat; Granola cereal; Pumpernickel bread; Oat bran muffins; Rice cakes (Brown rice based); Tortillas (corn); Chinese chow Mein noodles; Toasted bread;

Dairy Products, Fats & Oils

Chocolate milk; Milk (determine if milk & dairy products cause problems for your Ulcers); Cream cheese; Goat cheese; Cream; Whipped cream; Cheese: Gjetost, Limburger, Roquefort; Cheese spread; various cheese; Sour cream; Butter; Animal fat; Sesame oil; Whey (dried); Oils: coconut, Cupu Assu, Shea nut, tea seed, Ucuhuba Butter;

Instead choose: Margarine; Olive oil; Soybean oil;

Desserts, Snacks, Beverages

Chocolate ice cream; Coffee liqueur; Hot chocolate; Sweet chocolate; Dark chocolate; Coffee; 80+ proof distilled alcoholic beverages; Whiskey; Chocolate mousse; Chocolate chip cookies; Crème de menthe; Piña colada; Plain tea; Pound cake; Butter cookies; Wine; Vanilla ice cream; Dessert toppings; various cookies; Chocolate cake; Gingerbread cake; Beer;

Instead ***choose:*** ***Peanut butter; Sesame crunch candies; Tortilla chips; Peanut bar; Water; Halvah; Potato chips;***

Herbs & Spices, Fast Foods, Prepared Foods

Cocoa; Chocolate syrup; Cheese sauce; Horseradish; Mustard seed (avoid only if bothers you); Nutmeg (avoid only if it bothers you); Pepper (avoid only if it bothers you); Table sugar (white or powder); Nachos; Foie gras or liver pate;

Instead ***choose:*** ***Miso; Rosemary (fresh); Peppermint; Sweet pickle; Fried tofu; Pickle (cucumber); Spearmint (fresh); Tomato paste; Cloves; Oregano; Soy sauce; Cardamom; Croutons; Mayonnaise; Poppy seed; Sage; Sauerkraut; French salad dressing;***

Alternative Therapies & Miscellaneous

Aspirin (& other NSAID drugs); Fasting (for a specific period); Prescription drugs; 2+ alcoholic drinks/day; Excess body weight; Food allergens (determine if food allergy causes problems for your Ulcers); Smoking, tobacco; Stress;

Key Nutrients & Herbal Medicines

Caffeine; Alcohol; Buckthorn (Herb); Guarana; Kola (cola); Mate;

References

All the material and suggestions presented in this book are based on the content available at PersonalRemedies.com. The primary sources used by that web site and therefore this book are US government sources such as:

- USDA (US Department of Agriculture) including USDA Dietary Guidelines for Americans, nutrition.gov and mypyramid.gov.
- NIH (National Institute of Health) including Office of Dietary Supplements (ods.od.nih.gov), and MedlinePlus Health Information – a service of National Library of Medicine and NIH, National Diabetes Information Clearinghouse (NDIC), National Heart, Lung and Blood Institute ...
- Other organizations such as: Centers for Disease Control and Prevention (cdc.gov), National Cancer Institute (cancer.gov), US Environmental Protection Agency ...

For complete and detailed information about all the references please visit PersonalRemedies.com.

For Additional Information

For personal food list suggestions for

- other health conditions,
- other combinations of health conditions,
- a greater list of food choices, and
- for more detailed nutritional information,

you may wish to look at other books in our *Choose this not that* series listed on the last page or visit PersonalRemedies.com.

Acknowledgements

We would like to thank the following individuals for their support, encouragement, advice and contributions to the production of this book and contents of the Personal Remedies knowledgebase which is presented in this book: Ester Awnetwant-Esperon, MS, RD, LD; Karen Chiacu-Recco; Kate Fletcher-King; Amanda King; Avirat Kulkarni; Barbara Langathianos; Andrew Lenhardt, MD; Sih Han Lim; Mark Lu, MD; Steve Manson; Art McCray; Dick Neville; Christian Seeber; Nancy Elizabeth Shaw; Diana Silk; Scott Silk; George Sprenkle; Shahin Tabatabaei, MD; Foad Vafaei; Rolie Zagnoli; Mory Bahar.

Personal Remedies, LLC

and

Simple Software Publishing

Who is Personal Remedies?

Personal Remedies is a leading provider of knowledgebase & software for nutrition and health. The company can enable organizations such as hospitals, clinics, physician groups, food retailers, weight loss companies, leading fitness organizations, mobile phone operators and progressive corporations to provide consumer-centric nutrition, diet and health information tailored to the unique profile and goals of an individual.

Who is Simple Software Publishing?

Simple Software Publishing is a small publisher established in 1996. Our passion is to explain complex matters in an easy to understand form. We also strive to minimize the use of paper for production and distribution of books.

Choose this not that Series of Books, eBooks and Apps

- *Choose this not that* for **Breast Cancer**
- *Choose this not that* for **Cancer Prevention**
- *Choose this not that* for **Cervical Cancer**
- *Choose this not that* for **Colon Cancer**
- *Choose this not that* for **Esophageal Cancer**
- *Choose this not that* for **Gout**
- *Choose this not that* for **High Blood Pressure**
- *Choose this not that* for **High Cholesterol**
- *Choose this not that* for **High Triglycerides**
- *Choose this not that* for **Lung Cancer**
- *Choose this not that* for **Ovarian Cancer**
- *Choose this not that* for **Pancreatic Cancer**
- *Choose this not that* for **Prostate Cancer**
- *Choose this not that* for **Rheumatoid Arthritis**
- *Choose this not that* for **Stomach Cancer**
- *Choose this not that* for **Ulcers**
- *Choose this not that* for **Vitamin D Deficiency**
- *Choose this not that* for ... **please send us your suggestion!**

How to Order

To order eBooks (on Kindle or Nook) or printed copies of this book, or to order any of our other books please visit Amazon.com, Barnes & Noble, or contact us by email at Publisher@PersonalRemedies.com or send your purchase order or payments to:

> Simple Software Publishing
> 5 Oregon Street
> Georgetown, MA 01833

To order a colorful Mobile App version of this book, please visit Google Play Store (Android), or visit Amazon App Store.

For suggestions for new books and comments please email us at Books@PersonalRemedies.com.

Progress Tracker

To monitor your progress, date and note your symptoms and relevant data such as pain, pain-causing foods, blood pressure, weight, cholesterol level … below. We love to hear about your feedback and progress. Email us at Books@PersonalRemedies.com.

Notes

Made in the
USA
Monee, IL